The P

A science backed eating plan for reversing symptoms through restored hormone balance, increased fertility, and effective weight loss!

Jane Kennedy

Sandi,

this book gave me a lot of guidance and hope when it came to my PCOS. But even if there's only one bit of info that's applicable to your journey, I say it's worth the read!

♡ Jazz

The PCOS DIET

Jane Kennedy

Published by Jane Kennedy, 2019.

THE PCOS DIET

First edition. October 6, 2019.

Written by Jane Kennedy.

Table of Contents

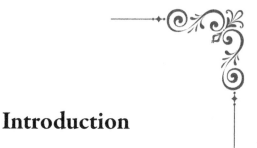

Introduction

Polycystic Ovary Syndrome (PCOS) is a troublesome syndrome that can cause life-altering symptoms that leave you feeling helpless and foreign to your own body. Depending on what form of PCOS you have, the symptoms can range from mild to extreme.

At first, you may not know you have PCOS. You miss a period and then it comes back heavier or maybe even lighter. The weeks between your periods start to get longer and longer. Then you notice that you're losing hair on your head. But, at the same time, you're growing hair on your upper lip, chin, and even in places on your body that you never had hair before. Out of nowhere, you get a severe case of acne. You feel 15 again, trying to get the acne to go away. If all these symptoms weren't bad enough, you begin to gain a lot of weight. It was a few pounds at first; but now, you've gained so much weight, you're having to buy new clothes.

These symptoms can go on for a time. Maybe you only have one or two of the symptoms I've described. Or maybe you have another symptom that I haven't mentioned yet: infertility. You've been trying to get pregnant and a year has gone by and still no baby. Not getting pregnant is the thing that finally takes you to your gynecologist. It's there that you first learn about

PCOS. You go in for tests hoping that you don't have PCOS, but in the end, you find out that yes, your symptoms and test results all point to the fact that you have PCOS.

You feel overwhelmed and confused about the treatment the doctor is suggesting. Treating PCOS requires more than just taking a or two pills. It requires something that is harder to achieve than most women want to admit – it requires a change of lifestyle.

In the United States, between 5-10% of women of child-bearing age have PCOS. It is the most common hormonal endocrine disorder in women and the most common cause of female infertility.

Along with a PCOS diagnosis comes frustration and fear. Yet, there are treatments that don't involve toxic medications or invasive procedures that take a toll on your body and spirit.

This book is about understanding PCOS and learning what you can do to become more active in your treatment. The symptoms of PCOS can be controlled. Whether through lifestyle changes, alternative supplements, or traditional prescribed medications, you can do something about PCOS.

After you meet with your doctor, it is important that you learn all you can about PCOS. What causes PCOS and what you can do about it, will probably be two of the most important questions that you can ask. Asking these questions are the first steps of your journey.

The next step of your journey is learning what you can do to be an active participant in your treatment. An effective treatment of PCOS is following a healthy diet. What you eat and how your body responds to your food are of paramount importance. Why? Hormonal imbalances are most likely the root cause of PCOS.

Too much of one hormone and not enough of another sets off a reaction that incites your body's endocrine system to go haywire. One of the direct effects of this chaos is the production of androgens that are responsible for many of the symptoms that you're experiencing. Researchers have found that insulin resistance is quite common in women with PCOS. Insulin resistance is your body's inability to deal with excess insulin.

Insulin resistance is not permanent. One way to stop insulin resistance is to eat complex carbohydrates that will not be absorbed as quickly as a simple carbohydrate. Is the answer as easy as swapping out your breakfast cereal with oatmeal? Well, not exactly.

Your body's digestive system is pretty complex, so it is going to take a combination of macronutrients to call to order a system that's gone wild. The easiest way to tackle this macronutrient issue is to follow a diet where carbohydrates, proteins and fats are delivered to the body in percentages that help your digestive system run properly.

Following a diet and staying on it are two extremely difficult things to do. Everyone has specific needs and habits. How do you know what diet will be sustainable for you but also good at getting your system to run properly? When your system is running properly, you will begin to see results and changes in your body and in the symptoms of your PCOS.

If you're feeling frustrated or scared because of a PCOS diagnosis or the symptoms you're experiencing, take comfort in knowing that a change in the way you eat has been shown to significantly improve common symptoms associated with poly-cystic ovarian syndrome and has often helped restore fertility to those afflicted with the condition.

Recent studies have found associations with a variety of macronutrients, supplements, and foods that can positively and negatively affect your PCOS symptoms. Due to the compli-cated nature of the causes behind each symptom, a diverse ap-proach should be taken when adjusting your eating habits to improve your condition.

This book takes a broad, all inclusive approach meant to be applied for women who are overweight, obese, or of nom-inal weight. The latest scientific data and personal experiences will be used to paint a complete picture of what healthy eating looks like for those of us with PCOS.

If fertility is your goal, know that many women who have been unable to conceive have reversed their infertility and en-tered motherhood due to healthy and positive changes in mindset, weight management, and diet!

For those who simply want to rid themselves of unwanted body hair, acne, or hair loss, the pages of this book will outline the dietary changes necessary to increase your chances of a re-duction or elimination of symptoms.

Note that this book will focus entirely on diet. There will be a separate, companion book available for those interested in looking into additional methods for reducing symptoms, but your DIET SHOULD NOT BE IGNORED, regardless of whether you have been diagnosed with PCOS.

Those with PCOS are looking for a way out, and many of us would like to explore options that don't include surgery or medication before we turn to such extreme measures. The good news is that thousands of women have recovered much of their natural hormone balance and fertility through positive changes and diet.

Continue reading to arm yourself with the information you need to be able to adjust your eating habits in a way that is sustainable long term, beneficial for your PCOS symptoms, and enjoyable.

The longer you wait before adopting your new lifestyle changes, the more the long-term symptoms of PCOS are going to set in.

Don't put off exploring the dietary information that you have available to you right here in this book any longer. Let's dive in!

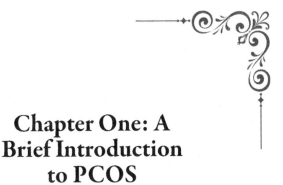

Chapter One: A Brief Introduction to PCOS

The year was 1991 and the National Institute of Health was trying to define a group of symptoms they saw over and over in women. In each case, the doctors repeatedly saw a critical hormonal imbalance. These hormone imbalances caused a myriad of conditions such as infertility, out of control hair growth and heavy weight gain.

The most the doctors could figure out was that there was something going on with the endocrine systems of the women they were treating. In each of these women, something was triggering a hormonal imbalance. Furthermore, these hormonal imbalances seemed to affect menstrual cycles and ovulation (Rose, 2014).

The doctors didn't think these symptoms belonged to any one particular illness. Young women of child bearing years and older, were showing the same groups of symptoms with slight variations. Moreover, each symptom had more than one cause. This being the case, the doctors decided that the symptoms they were seeing were part of a syndrome and not just one illness. Therefore, it became a syndrome with many symptoms that did not seem related to each other.

The syndrome that the doctors were treating came to be known as Polycystic Ovary Syndrome or PCOS. In an attempt to define PCOS, the Institute felt that three criteria had to be met. First, the patient had to show signs of a delayed period and, consequently, no ovulation. Second, there had to be an excess of hormones called androgens. And third, there had to be other conditions present that weren't part of any other illnesses.

The years passed and many more doctors began to treat women that seemed to have all the symptoms of PCOS and other metabolic issues that seemed to fit together. Consequently, in 2003 there was a meeting in the Netherlands between European and American health professionals to discuss this syndrome and the symptoms they were seeing in young women. Because the symptoms they were treating didn't fit the original criteria, they came up with the Rotterdam criteria. They decided that these three criteria had to be present in order to diagnose PCOS. Two of the criteria were the same as the original: delayed menstrual cycles with no ovulatution and the presence of excess androgens. The new third criteria they added was that polycystic ovaries had to be confirmed by ultrasound.

Then, those present at the meeting made a crucial decision: only two of the Rotterdam criteria had to be present in order for doctors to be able to diagnose PCOS. This was very different from the decision that was made at the National Health meeting.

Doctors began seeing more and more women who were infertile and desperate to have children, women who were suffering from internal inflammation, and women who were overweight and had symptoms of pre-diabetes because of insulin resistance. They diagnosed these women with PCOS. The symptoms of PCOS had gotten the attention of the medical research community and, consequently, research began in earnest because doctors were desperate to know how to treat the many young women who came in to their offices and were diagnosed with PCOS.

Facts About PCOS

Researchers soon determined that PCOS is not a disease. Ovaries may or may not develop cysts. Many PCOS patients are overweight and show signs of insulin resistance. PCOS is common in young women, and PCOS happens when there is an imbalance of hormones in a woman's body.

Understanding PCOS

To understand PCOS, it is important to recognize the many different symptoms. They have long scientific names that can be hard to understand. Let's break down the information into easy to understand chunks of information.

Anovulation

Anovulation means "lack of ovulation". This symptom is more than not ovulating. This term tells us that a woman diagnosed with anovulation has fewer periods per year than the average woman. Most women have a 29-day cycle. The start of the cycle is day 1, when your period starts, and then on day 14, you ovulate or release an egg and the cycle continues.

If one of your symptoms is Anovulation, it means that you have fewer than ten menstrual cycles per year, and consequently, you take more than 14 days to release an egg. It isn't just that your periods are long or short – it mainly means that you take so long to have a cycle, you have fewer periods during the calendar year.

Let us say that your period starts on day 1 and you have either a long or short period; yet after your period ends, you take longer than 14 days to release the next egg. In fact, it could take you more than thirty-five days or longer to release that egg and complete your cycle. Mathematically, because it takes you longer, you can't have more than 10 cycles a year. If you are trying to get pregnant, not having a cycle that is regular can really interfere with conception.

Anovulation is just one part of PCOS, and you don't have to be experiencing this symptom to have PCOS. However, anovulation is very common among women who are diagnosed with PCOS.

Excess Androgens

When the ovaries of women with PCOS release excess androgens, like testosterone, certain symptoms appear. These symptoms are called hirsutism. When you have hirsutism you have hair growth similar to a man's. A woman who has hirsutism may have hair on her chin, upper lip, nipples, chest, stomach, upper arms and thighs, or other areas. Another problem that is a result of excess androgens is severe or moderate acne along the jawline and back. If you don't have excess hair, you may develop hair loss that is similar to the way a man loses his hair. This is called hair loss in an androgenic pattern (androgenic means the development of male characteristics). The culprit of all of these symptoms are elevated hormones like DHEA and androstenedione.

Cysts and Follicles

Another symptom of PCOS that researchers had to define were the classification of the various kinds of cysts that are present in a woman with PCOS. The makeup of a cyst revolves around the number of follicles present.

When an ovary is healthy, the follicle goes through a growth cycle, known as folliculogenesis, many months before the egg is produced. But when the ovary is not healthy, and there is a high amount of testosterone in a woman's system, the outer layer of the follicle, the theca, grows thick and the growth of the follicle stops in its development process and accumulates in the ovaries rather than becoming an egg that is ready for fertilization.

Many of these follicles together make a cyst. The medical professionals that were attending the Rotterdam meeting in 2003 decided to clearly distinguish the cysts that were being found in PCOS. The determination was that there had to be twelve or more follicles with the size of two to nine millimeters in a single ovary. Furthermore, the ovary had to be bigger than ten centimeters. Plus, there had to be 26 follicles in the ovary (Briden, 2018).

Other cysts that are found in the body or around the ovary are different from the cysts found in PCOS. These other types of cysts are more complex than the cysts that are found in the ovary of a woman with PCOS. In fact, the PCOS cysts aren't really cysts when you compare them with these more complex cysts that contain blood or tissue and a large amount of fluid.

PCOS and its Phenotypes

PCOS is not an illness, disease, or condition. It is a syndrome which means that it is bigger than just one diagnosis. PCOS is a collection of diseases that are not linked to each other. In Rotterdam, the medical professionals defined different phenotypes that were associated with PCOS. A phenotype is "the set of observable characteristics of an individual resulting from the interaction of its genotype with the environment" (Brigham and Women's Hospital, 2015). The medical professionals defined four categories: Type A, Type B (classic PCOS), Type C, and Type D (not classic).

The Characteristics of the Different Phenotypes

The different phenotypes or classifications of PCOS were defined by the symptoms that the women displayed. The medical professionals classified PCOS into different categories in order to find effective treatments for these women. Type A patients had delayed ovulation, hyperandrogenism and polycystic ovaries on an ultrasound. Type B patients had delayed ovulation, hyperandrogenics, and normal ovaries on ultrasound. Type C patients had hyperandrogenics, with polycystic ovaries on ultrasound, and regular ovulation. And, type D patients had delayed ovulation with polycystic ovaries on ultrasound, without androgenic signs.

Patient Examples

Let's break down the different phenotypes into their unique characteristics. I will use patient examples to make things easier, because it can get confusing.

Anne has the type A phenotype, so she has a lack of ovulation and she does not have a 29 day cycle. In fact, she has less than 10 cycles happening per year. She also has hyperandrogenic symptoms which means that she may struggle with facial hair on her lip and chin. She might be insulin resistant or suffer from alopecia (hair loss). She also has polycystic cysts in her ovaries (PCO).

Barbra is type B phenotype and she has everything that Anne has, but she does not have PCO (cysts in her ovaries).

Carol has type C phenotype and she has the male-like hair growth on her body because she has high levels of testosterone and DHEA. She has regular cycles, but she has PCO.

Dana does not have to deal with the male pattern hair growth, but instead, she deals with her ovaries not releasing eggs for more than 10 months out of the year. She also has PCO

Not in Agreement

The medical community cannot agree on the phenotypes of PCOS. There is the international organization Androgen Excess and PCOS Society that believes excess androgens (hormones like testosterone) must be present for it to be a phenotype of PCOS. In other words, they do not believe that there should be a phenotype that does not show the symptoms of hyperandrogenism: hirsutism (excess facial or body hair), persistent acne and/or oily skin, alopecia (thinning hair on the head), insulin resistance, acanthosis nigricans (rough, darkly pigmented areas of skin), and high blood pressure.

Disorders That Mimic PCOS

It is interesting to note that there are other conditions and disorders that seem to present like PCOS, but they do not have all of the symptoms that form the PCOS syndrome. Here are some examples: Hypothyroidism is when the thyroid gland does not make enough thyroid hormones that the body needs. In this disorder, the thyroid is underactive. This disorder has some similar symptoms to PCOS such as weight gain. High Prolactin levels, which is too much prolactin in the blood of women who are not pregnant. And hypothalamic amenorrhea, a disorder that stops menstruation for months, so it is sometimes confused with PCOS.

What Pcos Is Like for Different Women

Each woman with PCOS needs to be treated differently and according to the symptoms that they are having, since PCOS manifests itself in different ways. The factors that affect PCOS types are age, weight, environment, genetics, and socio-emotions.

Sometimes a woman goes to the doctor to be treated for one of the symptoms of PCOS, like infertility, and she finds out that she has insulin resistance or high blood pressure. Another woman with PCOS who is being treated for cysts can find out that she has high cholesterol levels and is at risk for uterine cancer. These symptoms are part of the PCOS diagnosis, but they are not usually identified prior to diagnosis.

The Risk Factors

Not only do women with PCOS have to deal with a myriad of symptoms, but they are at risk for other illnesses. Women diagnosed with PCOS have: three times the risk of diabetes, stroke, and heart disease. Twice the risk for depression, drug use and anxiety. Twice the risk of hospitalization for any cause, and 10 times the risk of infertility (Raman, 2017).

PCOS and Infertility

80% of women that are diagnosed with PCOS are infertile because they do not have regular periods, and therefore they do not ovulate as much as a woman without PCOS. This is called anovulatory infertility. The first line of treatment for infertility is for a woman to change her lifestyle. For example, there is nutritional counseling to help a woman find a diet that may help her lose weight. The reason a woman with PCOS has to lose weight is that she may have insulin sensitivity which results in too much insulin in her bloodstream. Moreover, this increase in insulin causes the ovaries to produce more androgens. Increased androgens in her system causes irregular menstrual cycles.

Part of losing weight is going on a diet that can reverse insulin sensitivity. When insulin sensitivity or resistance is reversed, a woman with PCOS will have a better chance of ovulating regularly. Women with PCOS do not have to go through major weight loss for there to be an improvement to their menstrual cycles. Losing as little as 5-10% of body weight has been shown to have positive results (Galen, 2019).

The next line of treatment for infertility is medication. Clomid is a fertility drug that is used to treat patients with PCOS because it triggers ovulation. Not all women have success with Clomid because they can develop a resistance to it. Letrozole is a cancer medication that has been found to help increase fertility.

If Clomid or Letrozole are not successful, Gonadotropins (that are made up of FSH or LH or both hormones) are injected into your system. Often, a combination of oral and injectable medications are used to promote conception.

This kind of treatment is more successful when administered by a specialist who is familiar with PCOS.

Diet and Exercise Can Help Reduce Symptoms

Diet and exercise are particularly important because these lifestyle changes help correct insulin resistance and helps PCOS patients lose weight. A diet low in carbs and food that is of the highest nutritional quality is recommended (McCulloch, 2016). Also, the drug Metformin may be prescribed. Taking Metformin can help PCOS patients lose weight as it treats insulin resistance. Research has noted that Metformin also helps to regulate a PCOS patient's cycle.

Evidence to Eliminate PCOS

Today, there is evidence that there are many things a woman with PCOS can do to improve her condition and even eliminate some of the symptoms. The critical issue is to get the women who have PCOS diagnosed so they can begin healing. Often, an understanding of PCOS and a change of lifestyle can decrease the symptoms that a woman is experiencing.

If you suspect you have PCOS, being able to distinguish what type of PCOS you have can help you figure out what kind of changes you need to make in your lifestyle. In particular, you may have to make the decision to no longer smoke, drink alcohol, or do anything that can interfere with your healing.

It is important to see a doctor that understands PCOS and who can guide you into adapting a lifestyle that will help you eliminate some of the symptoms. In this book, we will be talking about diet and exercise, and the role each has in the healing of PCOS.

While this book focuses exclusively on diet and was written for those who wish to optimize their eating habits for their condition or lose weight, I have also written a companion piece covering all the treatment methods unrelated to diet. "PCOS, The New Science of Completely Reversing Symptoms," by myself, Jane Kennedy, is also available where you purchased this book.

CHAPTER SUMMARY

- PCOS is not a disease but a syndrome of many different symptoms.
- There are four different categories of PCOS.
- Lifestyle changes may reverse the symptoms of PCOS.

In the next chapter, you will learn about insulin resistance.

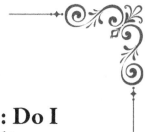

Chapter Two: Do I Have Insulin Resistance?

P COS doesn't happen to you without a cause. In this chapter, we will learn how insulin resistance affects your ovaries. In particular, when the body produces too much insulin, this triggers the ovary to produce more androgens, and this leads to critical symptoms of PCOS.

Being Overweight

The most common misconception about being overweight is that the reason you have the extra pounds is you don't have control over your appetite and therefore eat more calories than you can burn. While it is true that weight gain is caused by not burning enough calories from the food you eat leading whatever is left-over to become fat, there may be another factor contributing to your weight gain. In fact, you could have one of the symptoms of PCOS called insulin resistance.

The Key

Our body burns glucose for energy, but this glucose does not arrive to our cells on its own. To reach the cells that need this energy, glucose needs a key, and that key is insulin. Insulin is secreted by the pancreas when our blood sugar level rises.

Anytime we eat a food that is high in carbs and is high on the glycemic index, our blood sugar rises.

The Conversion of Carbs

The ideal situation for your body is to have a balanced meal where there isn't a substantial amount of carbs to accompany the fat and protein on your plate. Why? Carbs get converted into glucose and flood your body with sugar. The pancreas secretes insulin and tries to keep up with the glucose that is trying to get into your cells. If you eat a balanced meal, your blood sugar is moderately low, and your pancreas can keep up with your insulin production.

The Perfect Metabolic Process

This metabolic process is perfection in the way that cells are unlocked by insulin to let the glucose in. The cell takes the glucose and uses it, or if there is more than enough energy, the cell stores it. When your metabolic system is working properly, you maintain a healthy blood sugar level and everything is a go – meaning your cells are sensitive enough to maintain that healthy blood sugar level and the energy that is converted from glucose will be available when your body needs it.

The Liver and Its Role in the Metabolic Process

Another organ involved in the metabolic process is the liver. The liver stores glucose. The stored glucose is called glycogen, and it can be converted into energy whenever we need it. When the liver is functioning without stress, your body is running well. Your liver saves up the energy as glycogen, and releases it when you need more energy. Ideally, the glycogen is stored in your liver and muscles and released when you exercise.

Unresponsive Cells

In some women with PCOS, the metabolic process does not run well and they develop insulin resistance. This occurrence of insulin resistance happens in 70-95% of women with PCOS who are obsese and 30-75% of women with lean PCOS (Briden, 2018).

Insulin resistance means that cells do not respond to the insulin in your bloodstream, and when this happens, glucose stays in your bloodstream. The key no longer works, and the cells don't open up. Sensing that additional keys are needed to open up extra cells, the pancreas sends more insulin into your system. This is not good because not only do you have a high amount of blood sugar in your bloodstream, but you also have a high amount of insulin. This excess insulin will become a big problem to your system.

Working Overtime

The pancreas will go on producing as much insulin as it can, but over time, the pancreatic cells die and there is no longer insulin production in the body. When this happens, you have diabetes. But before you lose the ability to produce insulin, your body goes through what is called insulin resistance. When you have insulin resistance, no matter how many carbs you eat, excess blood sugar is in your system as if you have eaten a large high carb meal. Without the cells opening up to insulin, you are doomed to have too much insulin in your bloodstream.

The Consequence of Producing Too Much Androgen

How does this connect with PCOS? Remember that a feature or criteria of PCOS is an excess of hormones, specifically androgens. When there is a high level of insulin in your system, your ovaries produce more androgens, and this causes the body to have an excess of male hormones. The overload of androgens (testosterone) can interfere with your menstrual cycle, delay ovulation, and cause infertility.

Another result of excess androgens is hirsutism or hair on the chin, upper lip, and other parts of the body where hair doesn't usually grow on women. Androgens are mostly known as being male hormones and produce characteristics like excess body hair, male pattern baldness, and severe acne.

Good News

There is good news for women with PCOS, specifically women that are insulin resistant and are not yet diabetic. It is possible to eliminate some of your PCOS symptoms by eating a diet low in simple carbohydrates to stop an insulin overload and therefore keep the ovaries from making excessive amounts of androgens. When this happens, it is possible to get your menstrual cycle and ovulation back on track, as well as stop the other symptoms that happen as a result of too much androgen.

Testing for Insulin Resistance

To know if you are insulin resistant, you need to be tested. There are various kinds of testing to see how your body handles insulin. It isn't as simple as: if you are obese or overweight, you have insulin resistance. Moreover, if you are not obese, you can not assume that insulin resistance is not a problem for you.

When your doctor suspects that you may have insulin resistance as a symptom of PCOS, there are three different tests that he or she can give to you. The tests and calculations that are available to check for insulin resistance are:

- Fasting Insulin and Fasting Glucose Test – This test measures a ratio of insulin and glucose.

- The Insulin-Glucose Challenge Test – This test can pick up insulin resistance at the first sign of it occurring in your body.

- The HBA1C – This test measures blood glucose over a span of two to three months.

- The (HOMA-IR) that can be calculated to reveal if there is any insulin resistance.

Symptoms That Point to Insulin Resistance

Besides taking tests, there are other ways to figure out if you are insulin resistant (Roland, 2017). **Extreme hunger or thirst.** When you have this sign, you are unable to quench your thirst or satisfy your appetite. In fact, after you eat, you feel a gnawing hunger. **Eating a lot of snacks between meals** could indicate that you are not achieving satiety and feeling full enough after you eat. In fact, you may become shaky, dizzy, and feel like you need to have a snack in order to recover. **Tingling sensations in your hands and feet** is a sign of paresthesia. This happens when you damage your nerves and blood vessels with high blood sugar levels. **Frequent urination or polyuria** happens when you have a high blood glucose and your body needs to get rid of the excess glucose. **Acanthosis nigricans** is a skin condition that can be seen as dark patches in armpits or the back of your neck

These are only some signs of insulin resistance. It is important to see your doctor so that they can recommend tests that you should take to determine if you have insulin resistance.

Changing Your Eating Habits

If you find out you have insulin resistance, the first thing that your doctor will ask you to do is change the way that you eat. Consuming too many simple carbs can cause your body to convert the food too quickly into glucose, and this floods your bloodstream with too much blood sugar and overworks your pancreas to produce insulin. At the point of insulin resistance, you must help out your pancreas by not creating too much work for it. If there is less blood sugar in your system, the pancreas won't flood your body with insulin.

Insulin and PCOS

As discussed in chapter one, there are four different types of PCOS. Moreover, all of these types, except for one, have hyperandrogenic components to them: acne, excessive hair growth, hair loss, pimples, etc. All the types except for one includes anovulation, the lack of ovulation as a symptom. This lack of ovulation and hyperandrogenic components is related to too much insulin production and insulin resistance.

It stands to reason that in all of the different types of PCOS, insulin resistance plays a part, causing the ovaries to produce androgens in excess. Therefore, it is imperative that insulin resistance be treated. And, the most effective way to treat insulin resistance is to change your diet. Many women have been able to reverse some of their PCOS symptoms and increase fertility and regulate their ovulation cycle by changing their diet and lifestyle (McCulloch, 2016). Taking measures to get back insulin sensitivity is key to overcoming PCOS.

Later in this book, I will delve into the impact of diet on PCOS, and I will detail what kinds of foods you can eat to help get you out of insulin resistance. I will also talk about lifestyle changes, such as exercise, that will help your body reverse the effects of PCOS. But for now, I will summarize the diets that we will discuss in this book.

Diets That Can Help with Insulin Resistance

A low carb diet can help insulin resistance by introducing into the diet more proteins and eating complex carbohydrates. The amount of carbs in your diet has a direct correlation to the level of blood sugar in your body.

In this book, we will learn about the glycemic index and how you can use your knowledge about the amount of carbs in your meals to your advantage. The glycemic index is an index that ranks foods from 1-100. Foods low on the index have little effect on your blood sugar and foods high on the index markedly affect your blood sugar and should be avoided.

The Keto Diet

The keto diet helps to lower your blood sugar level by inducing your body to burn more fat. Instead of producing more glucose by eating carbs, you eat an exceptionally low amount of carbs to prompt your muscles to release glycogen that your body can burn for energy. Furthermore, you eat more fat and protein to help keep your blood glucose down. In fact, you change the way that your body gets its energy by putting your body into a state of ketosis.

When your body doesn't have enough glucose to burn for energy, it forces the body to burn stored fat. When this happens, there are acids called ketones that are released into your body. This diet lowers your blood sugar so that your pancreas does not have to work so hard in producing insulin. Following this diet can help reverse insulin resistance.

The PCOS Diet

The PCOS diet is more a way of life and making good choices like regularly drinking enough water, eating complex carbohydrates, and managing your diet to control the amount of blood sugar in your bloodstream. The PCOS diet is similar to the keto diet in the way that it counts macronutrients such as carbohydrates, proteins and fats, but it does not encourage decreasing your carb intake and eating more protein. Another difference is, in the PCOS diet there is no emphasis on fasting or putting yourself into a ketogenic state so that your body will release glycogen into your bloodstream and burn it for energy instead of glucose.

PCOS and Insulin Resistance

PCOS can be a difficult syndrome to deal with, but you have it in your control to change some of the things that trigger it. There are different types of PCOS, but all of them share insulin resistance as a cause. Too much insulin and high blood sugar signals the ovaries to produce androgens such as testosterone. This production of androgen leads to symptoms like hyperandrogenism and anovulation. A healthy diet and exercise can help reverse insulin resistance.

Chapter Summary

- Insulin resistance is behind many symptoms of PCOS.

- A diet of simple carbohydrates causes too much insulin to be released into the bloodstream.

- Diet and lifestyle changes can reverse some of the symptoms of PCOS.

In the next chapter, you will learn about exercise as a lifestyle change.

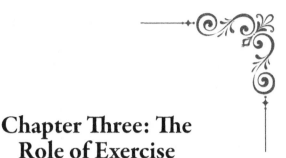

Chapter Three: The Role of Exercise

According to the American Diabetes Association, "working out can increase your cells' response to insulin and allow them to more easily use glucose for energy" (Mayo Clinic Staff, 2019).

In a body that is wrecked from a hormonal imbalance, there is a craving to be healthy and balanced. Women with PCOS need interventions to help them with the symptoms that are challenging and compromising their well-being.

More and more women are becoming sedentary because of their work or perhaps because they don't feel well enough to be active. PCOS can be triggered by a life of no activity and poor eating habits.

If you are a person that already has a routine of exercise, you know that movement and aerobic exercise is especially important. It takes commitment and a strong will to get out there and exercise when you may not be feeling good about yourself. PCOS isn't debilitating like other syndromes or diseases, but it does interfere with the functions of your body. If you do not exercise regularly, today is the best time to start.

Being Sedentary and PCOS

Being sedentary is not good for your PCOS. If you do not exercise, you will not have the chance to burn more energy. Activating the energy reserves in your liver and your muscles is very important. When you need more energy, your liver and muscles release glycogen and your body uses glycogen for more energy. When this happens, you need less insulin and therefore less insulin is produced. Consequently, your ovaries will not release androgens because there is no excess insulin to activate them.

Exercise Guidelines

The "Evidence Based Guideline for Assessment and Management of PCOS", published in the Medical Journal of Australia, offered some exercise guidelines to help women with PCOS. These guidelines recommended that women exercise for 150 minutes per week and that at least 90 minutes of the 150 minutes should be moderate to strenuous aerobic activity.

It might be exceedingly difficult for you to do this. If you suffer from insulin resistance, you are dealing with other issues such as insomnia or feeling fatigue. Since you feel ill, it might be hard to believe that getting more active can help you get over the symptoms that are keeping you from enjoying your best life.

Starting Slow

You don't have to qualify for the Olympics on your first time out. Perhaps you feel that joining a health club might be too much for you. Don't worry, you can start exercising at home or even in your backyard. Simple isometric exercises that do not cost anything can be done anywhere. Keeping it simple and going slow is a good way to start. Some examples of the isometric exercises you can do from home on your own are bicep curls, toe raises, walking lunges, deep squats, and toe touches.

After you do these isometric exercises, you can enjoy a brisk walk for twenty minutes. The amount of exercise that you do is up to you. Start with 6 to 10 reps and work up to 20-30 reps. These types of exercises can be done for a prolonged period of time and can ease you into having an exercise regime.

The purpose of exercise is to burn off some energy and get your cells responding to insulin again. If your cells do respond, the pancreas doesn't have to work so hard and your cells can start functioning again. This happens because you exercised and called on your body to exert itself.

Paying Attention to Your Heart

Your reaction to exercise can be mixed. At times, it might feel like you do not want to leave your chair or sedentary way of life. You might feel awkward about doing anything physical. Other days, you might be highly motivated to start an exercise regimen so that you can reverse the symptoms of PCOS. The most important thing to do when you start exercising is to pay attention to your heart.

You goal when you exercise is to raise your heartbeat from a normal resting level. You want your exercise program to be moderate to high intensity, and the way to gage whether your body is reaching that level is to have a target heart rate. The goal is to raise your heart beat to a 50% to 90% heart rate.

Here is a formula you can use to determine what your target heart rate should be:

220 - your age = maximum heart rate

So, for example, I am 34, so my formula would look like this:

220-34= 186

One hundred eight-six is the average maximum number of times my heart should beat per minute during exercise Orlov, 2017). If I want my target rate to be 50% of my average maximum heart beat, I would use this equation 0.50 x 186 = 93. 93 would be my target pulse rate.

To use this formula to increase my exercise from moderate to vigorous, I would multiply by 70% or even 85% instead of 50%.

It is important to get in the habit of exercise because it can be a game changer in your struggle with PCOS. More women who make lifestyle changes have found relief from the symptoms of PCOS than women who do not. So, it is in your best interest to choose exercise as a way to heal yourself (Orlov, 2017).

Moving Beyond Your Starting Point

Isometrics is a nice way to start, but to get to your target heart rate, you will want to do cardio exercises. Here is a list of cardio exercises that you might enjoy:

Swimming Cycling

Jumping Rope Zumba

Skipping rope Jogging

Belly Dancing Tennis

Yoga Hiking

CrossFit training Hiking

Don't be afraid of raising your heart rate and doing cardio exercises. The more often you reach your target heart rate, the better you will feel. In fact, you may begin to see and feel that some of your PCOS symptoms disappear entirely.

Exercises That Raise Your Metabolic Rate

When you exercise, you raise your metabolic rate. But first, let's go over what the basal metabolic rate or BMR is:

"BMR is the number of calories your body needs for basic body functions that keep you alive, such as your heartbeat, breathing and the regular upkeep of your body organs; it's essentially the number of calories you need if you did nothing but lie around all day" (Corleone, 2019).

When you know this number, you can begin to make a strategy for weight loss or any other goals you might have.

The equation to use is the Mifflin St Jeor Equation (Orlov, 2017).

For men: BMR = 10 x weight (kg) + 6.25 x height (cm) – 5 x age (years) + 5

For women: BMR = 10 x weight (kg) + 6.25 x height (cm) – 5 x age (years) – 161

For example:

BMR = 10x154(kg) + 6.25 x 162.6 (cm) - 5 x 54 (years) -161

BMR = 1540 + 1016 - 270 - 161

BMR = 2556 - 270

BMR = 2286 - 161

BMR = 2125

Putting Your BMR to Work

Now that you know your BMR, what do you do with this number? Why is it important?

Well, now you know how many calories it takes for your body to function. To lose weight, you need to eat fewer calories. For example, to lose 1 pound a week, you'd reduce your calorie intake by 500 calories.

The Activity Factor

Your BMR number will decline has you get more fit because your resting heart rate will get lower. Specifically, your heart will be working more efficiently. Your body moves according to your needs. You may be a very active person or maybe you are a person who loves to sit and observe life. There are activity numbers that impact your BMR too.

According to LIVESTRONG.COM, this is a list of numbers you can use to determine the number of calories that you burn through daily activities based on your overall activity level:

Use 1.2 if you lead a sedentary life.

Use 1.375 if you exercise three to five days a week.

Use 1.55 if you exercise six to seven days a week.

Use 1.725 if you are involved in sports and exercise six to seven times a week.

Use 1.9 if you are training for a marathon or have a physically challenging job.

Here's an example of how to update your BMR with your activity level from LIVESTRONG.COM:

For a 41-year old woman with a BMR of 1,388 calories and an activity number of 1.375, the equation would look like this:

1388 x 1.375 = 1,908.5

Subtract 500 calories, and that leaves 1,409 calories a day to lose 1 pound a week.

Exercise That Challenges You

Weight training is one of the best ways to exercise. Free weights may be the best, but you can also use exercise machines. A trainer can show you how to use the weight machines and how to adjust the weights for your level. Weight training every other day is ideal to help defeat insulin deficiency.

Digital Help

If doing the math is complicated for you, there are BMR calculators on websites and apps for your smartphone or tablet. There are also websites with the BMR calculator. Just use the keyword BMR calculator to find them.

These websites can help you to determine your body fat or BMI (body mass index), caloric needs, BMR, nutritional needs, ideal weight, heart rate, and running pace.

Before you start an exercise program, see your doctor to get the all clear.

PCOS and Losing Weight

Not all women who have PCOS need to lose weight. In fact, losing weight isn't meant to be the focus of your new healthy lifestyle. The most important thing is that you get your blood sugar levels down to a level that helps the cells and insulin function properly.

There are many other goals that you want to reach, like being able to use your body the way it was meant to be used. For example, walking is beneficial because it helps you to build stamina. The more stamina that you have, the more you will be able to exercise. The more you exercise, the more weight you will lose, and the more weight you lose, the more efficient your body becomes at releasing insulin and burning energy. When this happens, you will no longer be insulin resistant.

Weight That Won't Come Off

When you have PCOS, your hormones are imbalanced, and that may affect your ability to lose weight. There is a theory that what you weigh is a factor of genetics, hormones and neurotransmitters, plus our life experiences with food (Orlov, 2017). It is also believed that you will remain at the weight that you have been for a period of time. You may go on diets and lose weight, but you will eventually return to the weight you were at the longest.

It is very difficult to lose weight if you are a woman with PCOS. It is not impossible, but you have to be patient with yourself and understand your situation. You have hormones that are not balanced and you may have insulin resistance – all these things can be turned around by exercise.

Keep the Faith

Even though your goal may be to lose weight, you don't have to lose a great amount to help your PCOS. You just need to get your body functioning as it should, and this will come in stages. Remember that the point of exercise isn't to become super thin but to lower your blood sugar and once you do that, you may be able to stop the progression of PCOS.

Weeks 1-2

Start slowly, and do something you enjoy for small periods of time. Short bursts of ten minutes each is better than doing nothing at all. If you are already an active person, do an activity like tennis or swimming that you totally enjoy. But engage in it slowly and carefully if it has been a long time since you've been active. This week is about taking it slow.

If you have a smart watch or a smartphone, you can keep track of your steps and heart rate. Set small goals, and try to reach them. Try to stay at your target for five to ten minutes and concentrate on how it feels. Focus on parts of your body that have not been active in a long time. Even if you were once a star athlete, it is good to get reacquainted with your body again before pushing it too far.

Weeks 3-4

Walking can be enjoyed with your partner or a friend. Just walk for fun, and try to walk a little further every day. Take small steps and be mindful of your body. Do some stretching exercises when you start walking further. If you have a smart watch or a smartphone, utilize it fully to count your steps and measure distance.

Weeks 5-6

This is the week that you pick up speed when you walk. If you are an active or semi-active person, it is time to get that aerobic exercise done. Pick an activity like swimming, or you can continue walking. The goal here is to pick up speed. You might buy some good running shoes and pick an activity that challenges you.

First, you stretch a little bit before you start your run or walk. Then walk or jog at a slow pace to warm up. When you are warmed up, take a brisk walk for one minute and then go back into slower walk for 5 minutes; and then, walk home and stretch. If you have already been walking, it's okay to work a little harder to get a good work out.

In the future, you will develop other exercise routines that are fun for you. Perhaps you love the indoors and prefer a gym where you can work out with other people. If you are a shy soul, pick a small, private nook, away from the crowds.

Join the Crowd

After six weeks you are probably feeling better than you ever have before. You may want to join a class. Some classes that you could join are: yoga, pilates, tai chi, Zumba, silver sneakers, and yes, even spin class. As you begin to be more comfortable, join a health club that offers you a variety of exercise options like circuit training, treadmills, swimming pools, walking/running tracks, and exercise classes.

Now that you are active, always respect your limits and don't push yourself too hard. See the doctor and run the tests again to see if your body is now out of insulin resistance. During these weeks, you may even begin to menstruate again and ovulate.

Turning PCOS Around

Exercise of any sort is very good for you. At first, it will be hard, but then you will find a happy medium and acquire the habit of exercise. Doing this can be a game changer in your struggle with PCOS.

Participating in Your Treatment

There are things you can do to fight the symptoms caused by hormone imbalances. Lifestyle changes can help reverse these symptoms. Changing your lifestyle is all about doing things that can make your body stronger and give you a sense of well-being. PCOS can have a big impact on your life; especially if you suffer from insulin resistance. It is important that you are in a doctor's care, but there are many things you can do to participate in your treatment.

Chapter Summary

- Exercise can reverse the effects of PCOS.
- Get tested to learn if you are insulin resistant.
- Start an exercise routine gradually, and work up to being more active.

In the next chapter, you will learn about androgens and their role in PCOS.

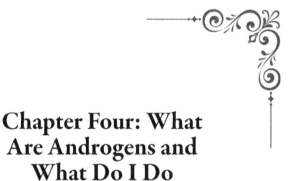

Chapter Four: What Are Androgens and What Do I Do About Them?

In Chapter Two, we established that too much insulin in the body triggers the ovary to produce androgens. But what exactly are androgens? Often referred to as the male hormone, androgens are responsible for reproductive function, lean muscle functions and growth, bone strength, emotional well-being, and cognitive functions (Gurevich, 2019).

There are various androgen hormones that affect our body. The following is a description of some of the androgens that affect a woman's body.

Testerone

Testosterone is found in both ovaries and the adrenals. But, 50% of testosterone comes from the conversion of androstenedione in the bloodstream (McCulloch, 2016).

When there is an excess amount of testosterone in a woman's body, she may develop frontal balding, an enlarged clitoris, a deep voice, and increased muscle mass (Gurevich, 2019).

DHEA

DHEA is secreted by the adrenal glands. Too much DHEA and you get oily skin and acne. You also have hair loss, but at the same time, you get facial hair. Your voice deepens and you are fatigued. DHEA is also a culprit in changing your menstrual cycle.

DHEA-s

DHEA-s is the most abundant hormone in your body when you are of reproductive age. It is produced by the adrenals. DHEA-s peaks in your early adulthood, and then the level goes down as you get older.

Androstenedione

Androstenedione is produced by the ovaries and the adrenals. This hormone in excess also causes excess body and facial hair, it may stop periods, and stimulate worsening acne.

Dihydrotestosterone

Dihydrotestosterone (DHT) is the most powerful androgen and is produced in the tissue of the body. DHT is responsible for hair loss.

What Androgens Do for Your Body

When androgens are balanced, they contribute a lot to your body. They are responsible for improving muscle mass, keeping your libido strong, and moderating body fat. Androgens are also necessary for bone, kidney and liver health, as well as fertility (McCulloch, 2016).

What Happens When There Are Too Many Androgens

When there are too many androgens, women experience "masculinization. Characteristics that are normally attributed to men, begin to appear in a woman's body. This includes the appearance of hair on the upper lip, chin, mid-chest, abdomen, and back. These are areas where you would find hair on a man.

If there is excessive hair on other parts of the body, androgens are not responsible for that, as they are just responsible for male attributes. An excess of androgens is the most common culprit of hirsutism (McCulloch, 2016).

An excess of androgens is also responsible for the condition called Androgenetic Alopecia (female-pattern hair loss). It is very stressful for women who begin to lose their hair. Too many androgens are responsible for this.

Ways to Correct Androgen Excess

There are medications that can help with androgen excess such as birth control pills and steroids. In this chapter, I will focus on the natural treatments of androgen excess. It's important at this point to know what the source of your adrenal excess is. You may have an excess of derived androgens (DHEA-S) or maybe you have ovarian androgens (testosterone) or perhaps you have a bit of both playing havoc with your system (McCulloch, 2016).

Natural therapies can help the symptoms of excess androgens such as hirsutism, acne, and androgenetic alopecia. If you have either type of androgen excess, as discussed above, natural therapies may be able to help you.

Licorice (Glycerrhiza glabra)

In a 2004 study, "Licorice Reduces Serum Testosterone in Healthy Women," researchers found that licorice significantly decreased testosterone levels in women after one month of treatment (McCulloch, 2016). The licorice blocks key enzymes involved in the making of testosterone. There are also some steroids in licorice (glycyrrhizin and glycyrrhetinic acid) that have anti-androgen effects (McCulloch, 2016). The anti-androgen effects have been shown to be helpful in reducing androgenetic alopecia, hirsutism, and acne in women with PCOS.

Please note that if you have high blood pressure, licorice has been shown to raise blood pressure, so you shouldn't try this natural remedy if you have hypertension.

White Peony (Paeonia Lactiflora)

White Peony is a popular anti-androgenic herb and often used in traditional Chinese medicine by combining it with licorice at a ratio of 1:1. The peony and licorice formula is given at a dosage of two grams, three times per day and up to four grams, three times a day (McCulloch, 2016).

White peony works by decreasing the creation of testosterone but does not alter the production of androstenedione and estradiol (McCulloch, 2016). The formula of white peony and licorice is given to help regulate the menstrual cycle and reduces androgenic signs like hirsutism and acne.

Tea

Both Spearmint and marjoram herb tea both have an impact on PCOS and hirsutism. Spearmint was tested by researchers who gave spearmint tea to women in a randomized study. The results published in *Phytotherapy Research* showed that free and total testosterone levels were reduced over the 30-day period in women who drank the tea twice a day. These women also felt that their hirsutism got better.

Spearmint tea isn't the only tea that has had an impact on PCOS. Women who drank marjoram tea twice a day for one month experienced improved insulin sensitivity and lower levels of adrenal androgens compared to the women who drank the placebo. This study was published in the *Journal of Human*

Nutrition. Marjoram herb tea also restored hormonal balance and regulated menstrual cycles in women.

Red Reishi Mushrooms

In a study of 20 distinct species of mushrooms, the red reishi mushroom was the species of mushroom that had anti-androgenic effects. Red Reishi is a Japanese mushroom that has many health benefits. The mushroom considerably decreases levels of 5-alpha-reductase that prevents the conversion of testosterone into the more powerful DHT. These decreased levels affect acne and baldness.

Flaxseed

Can one woman make a difference in the fight against PCOS? Yes, she can. A 31-year old woman with PCOS took 30 grams a day of flaxseed, and the results were a reduced total of free testosterone (Very Well Health). This woman also had a reduction in hirsutism at the end of the study. Men with prostate cancer have also reacted to flaxseed and experienced diminished androgen levels.

Nuts

Researchers have found that nuts have a beneficial effect on androgen levels in women with PCOS. In a study published in the European Journal of Clinical Nutrition, random women were chosen to take part in a study where they gave some women walnuts or almonds for six weeks. It turned out that the women who ate walnuts increased their levels of sex-hormone binding globulin (SHBG) and that the women who ate almonds had decreased free androgen levels (Very Well Health).

Fish

47.2% vs. 22.9% was the total of the effectiveness of omega-3 vs. placebo in a study that was published in *Iran Jour-*

nal of Reproductive Medicine. Seventy-eight overweight women with PCOS were randomly sorted - with one group receiving 3 grams of omega-3 per day, and the other half of the group receiving a placebo for eight weeks. In the end, it was seen that testosterone concentration was really low in the omega-3 group compared with the placebo group.

Other foods and natural sources that made a significant improvement to reduce androgens are black cohosh (phytoestrogen), saw palmetto, rosemary, melatonin, kudzu root, and iron.

Curing Acne

Some women who have an increase in androgens have trouble with acne. Certain topical treatments by natural sources has proven to be effective. Those sources are: salicylic acid, tea tree oil made from white willow bark, japanese cypress oil, and alpha hydroxy acids.

Choosing foods that are anti-inflammatory also helps. For example, tomatoes, olive oil, green leafy vegetables like kale, nuts like almonds, fatty fish like salmon and tuna, and fruits such as oranges, cherries, blueberries and strawberries can reverse some of the symptoms of PCOS (Harvard Health Publishing).

Androgen excess is an issue with women who have PCOS. The symptoms can be keeping ovulation from happening and delaying menstrual cycles. Moreover, some women will have excess hair growth and severe acne due to increased androgens. This being the case, there are natural alternatives and medication that can help women resolve the issues they have because of PCOS.

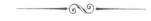

CHAPTER SUMMARY

- Increased androgens affects the body in distinct ways.
- There are medications to help decrease androgen levels.
- There are natural alternatives that decrease androgen levels.

In the next chapter, you will learn about the glycemic index.

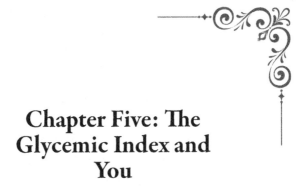

Chapter Five: The Glycemic Index and You

Part of the treatment for PCOS is to improve nutrition and deal with the insulin sensitivity connected to this syndrome. One of the best tools to use when trying to reverse the effects of insulin sensitivity is to know the glycemic index of foods that you are going to eat.

What is the Glycemic Index?

The glycemic index or GI tells you how your body reacts to a food. Specifically, the effect that the food has on your blood glucose levels. When you have a food that is high on the GI, this means that the food is quickly digested and metabolized, causing a rapid rise in your body of blood glucose. The amount of blood glucose in your body determines how much insulin your pancreas releases. A large amount of insulin will lead you to develop insulin sensitivity. As your insulin levels rise, so does the production of testosterone.

When a food has a low number on the glycemic index, this means it is digested and metabolized slowly, and there is a slow rise of blood glucose in your system. Insulin is secreted by your pancreas, which enables your cells to absorb blood glucose and make energy. Since the cells are absorbing the glucose, there is less in your bloodstream and the pancreas stops releasing insulin into your system. Consequently, with less insulin in your system, production of testosterone stays at a "normal" level.

PCOS and Testosterone

When dealing with PCOS, there tends to be a higher than normal production of testosterone. This is tied to a woman having insulin sensitivity and producing more testosterone. The glycemic index becomes especially important in the treatment of PCOS, because ideally, a woman should be eating foods that are low on the glycemic index so that she can reverse her insulin sensitivity.

The Glycemic Load

However, just knowing the glycemic index of a food is not enough to reverse insulin sensitivity. Women must also consider the Glycemic Load (GL) of a food. The glycemic load measures the amount of food that you are eating and its effect on your blood glucose levels. To find the glycemic load of a food, you must know the glycemic index. An equation to find the GL is as follows:

(Glycemic Index x grams of carbs)/100 = Glycemic Load

The Glycemic Load of a Donut

Here is an example of how you would figure out what the glycemic load of a donut is.

First, you look up the glycemic index of the donut. My list says that a donut's GI is 76. Now you look up the grams of carbohydrates in the donut. You can usually find this listed on the Nutritional Information section of the packaging. Let's say mine is 22 grams. Now let's plug those numbers into the above equation.

$(76 \times 22)/100 = 16.72$

Is the donut's glycemic load number high?

Let's look at the ranges:

1-10 is low.

11-19 is medium.

20+ is high.

Looks like the donut falls in the medium range for the glycemic load. However, do you ever just eat one donut? If you can eat just one, I really admire you. But if you're anything like me, and you can't stop at just one, consider how your body will absorb two donuts or a 33.44 glycemic load. Now we're in the high range, and for anyone with PCOS, such foods should be avoided.

Distinct Types of Carbohydrates

If you are unsure what foods are carbs and what foods aren't, let's look at some of the obvious and not so obvious carbohydrates. There are ten different types of sugars and each one of them reacts in the body in different ways. All of these sugars are of a class that can not be hydrolyzed into a simpler sugar. Here is a break down of these types of sugars and what foods have them.

Glucose (<u>monosaccharide</u>) is the body's main source of energy

Fructose (monosaccharide) is in honey, tree and vine fruits, berries, and root vegetables. Sugar cane, sugar beets, and maze make commercial fructose.

Galactose (monosaccharide) is found in dairy products, avocados, and sugar beets.

Sucrose (<u>disaccharide</u>) is found naturally in pineapples and apricots. It is found commercially in poultry and pork products, sausage and luncheon meats, fats and oils, and snacks.

Lactose (disaccharide) (milk sugar) can be found naturally in milk, yogurt, cream, butter, ice cream, and cheese. Commercially, it is found in pancake mixes, ready-to-eat breakfast cereals, instant soups, candy, cookies, and drink mixes.

Cellulose (polysaccharides) is the chemical name for fiber and is found in plants. It can not be digested by humans but it is really important that we eat cellulose/fiber. Fruits and vegetables have cellulose.

Chitin (a polysaccharide) is the main ingredient in exoskeletons of crustaceans and arthropods, but it is also present in mushrooms, shellfish, and escargots. It is used as a food thickener and stabilizer.

Starch is in bread, pasta, rice, couscous, potatoes, breakfast cereals, oats, and other grains. Starch is a polysaccharide that is made by combining a large number of glucose monomers together.

Xylose is a dietary sugar that is found in fruits, cereals, bread, and vegetables like potatoes, peas and carrots. Xylose is a sugar used as a diabetic sweetener in foods and beverages.

Maltose or malt sugar is present in malt products like malted milkshakes and malted candies, grains, and starchy vegetables. Maltose can also be found in foods where starch is fermented by yeast as in breads or brewed beverages.

These different types of sugars are good to know because all carbohydrates are not created equal. When we think of carbs, we think of bread, rice and pasta as a rule, but sugars can be found in other things. We try to not have too much of these foods because we are told that too much is not good for us. It is good to know, for example, that xylose is a sugar that can be tolerated by diabetics. Eating low carb seems to be the trend right now in weight loss, but we have to give pause to the different nutrients that come to us through carbohydrates or simple sugars.

The Glycemic Load of a Banana

It's hard to believe, but there are carbohydrates in foods that we need to eat for their nutritional value. Fruits and vegetables fall into the category of carbohydrates. Should we not eat a banana that has a glycemic index of 51?

Let's look at that equation for the glycemic load.

(Glycemic Index x grams of carbs)/100 = Glycemic Load

(51 x 27g)/100= 13.77

The glycemic load of a banana is in the medium range, so it isn't too bad, especially if we only have one banana.

What About Vegetables?

Potatoes, pumpkins, and sweet potatoes have a high glycemic index, but carrots, green beans, and plantains, just to name a few, are below 50. The sweet potato might be thought of as being healthier than a potato, because it is high in fiber, vitamin C, potassium, pantothenic acid, niacin, vitamin B6, manganese, magnesium, copper, and beta carotene. So, you see, not all carbs are bad for you and cutting them out completely may not be a good thing. That is why these diets are called low carb. You still need carbs in your diet, but you need to make these carbs count. So while vegetables like sweet potatoes may be high in carbs, they have other benefits that make them still worth eating in moderation.

Hidden Carbs

When you are concerned with insulin sensitivity, it is important to pay attention to the glycemic index and glycemic load so that you can get a handle on the amount of blood glucose you will have in your body.

While counting carbs, you must be incredibly careful of the hidden carbs in all foods. Some obvious sources of hidden carbs are in sauces or condiments like the following: ketchup, barbecue sauce, sriracha sauce, teriyaki sauce, and balsamic vinegar.

It was a trend for a while to drink juice instead of soft drinks, but although fruit drinks are natural, they have a lot of carbs. Apple juice for example has 28 g of carbs in one cup. There is a whole industry for promoting natural foods. So, read the label when you are picking something healthy. Remember, your goal is not to obliviate carbs, you are just trying to give your body a break when it comes to your pancreas releasing insulin. You are paying attention to the glycemic index and glycemic load so that you can give your body every chance to work properly and eliminate some of the symptoms of your PCOS

Sugars That Take Longer to Absorb

For an example of high glycemic load counts, we looked at the differences between a regular potato and a sweet potato. The sweet potato was packed with a lot of fiber, vitamins, and minerals. Keeping this in mind, think about refined sugar and processed flour.

In the morning, I have oatmeal that is protein enriched with a tablespoon of sugar. The glycemic index for this is low because the oatmeal has fiber and protein, so it takes longer to digest. And a tablespoon of sugar, isn't the best, but it isn't the worst either.

Compare this one tablespoon with the amount of sugar in a breakfast cereal. The USDA says that, on average, a breakfast cereal can have as much as 55 grams of carbohydrates in one cup (81 grams). One tablespoon of sugar has 13 grams of carbohydrates.

The more processed your food, the higher in carbs that food is going to be. The higher the carbs, the harder it will be for your body to metabolize those carbs into energy.

Why Does All This Matter for a Woman With Pcos?

We've discussed the connection between insulin sensitivity and the production of testosterone, which leads to androgen excess. But let's look at another factor: "Women with PCOS store fat more efficiently and burn up calories more slowly than women who don't have PCOS" (Harris & Francis-Cheung, 2016).

In other words, a woman who has PCOS may have a slower metabolism than a woman without PCOS. Not being able to lose weight like other women who do not have PCOS can be really frustrating. However, when you begin to follow a healthy diet and exercise, you can change your metabolism.

If your weight gain is significant, you are at risk for more health problems such as obesity, eating disorders, cholesterol problems, high blood pressure, and cardiovascular disease. It is important to do things to lose weight.

PCOS and Diabetes

One condition that a women with PCOS can have is non-insulin dependent diabetes. "A woman with PCOS is seven times more likely to develop diabetes during her lifetime than the rest of the populations" (Harris & Francis-Cheung, 2016). Whatsmore, if you have hyperinsulinemia and insulin resistance, your chances of developing gestational diabetes is greater. Although the diabetes will likely go away after you give birth, you are still at risk for diabetes in your future (Harris & Francis-Cheung, 2016).

Does this mean you will have a bleak future? Not at all, if you know that you have PCOS and one of the symptoms that you have is insulin resistance, you can change the odds by following a healthy diet.

Clinical nutritionist Conner Middleman Whitney, who studied nutrition and PCOS via "a three-month internet study involving dietary changes and nutritional supplements" concluded that nutritional therapy can offer "powerful support" (Harris & Francis-Cheung, 2016). In other words, you will be in good shape, if you follow a food plan and seek support through resources like a diet support group or a nutritionist. Just as long as you make nutrition a priority, you will make progress in your weight loss efforts.

Being Aware

In this book, we will discuss different diets that can be a game changer when it comes to PCOS. Being aware of the glycemic index and glycemic load is a particularly good start. Don't get overwhelmed with this awareness. A simple awareness of where a food fits into the glycemic index can be extremely helpful when you are planning your meals.

Watching what you eat is going to count a lot when it comes to reducing health risks and your PCOS. Eating healthy can go a long way in preventing illnesses like diabetes and infertility.

Examples of Low-Carb Dieting

Before you start a diet that will change your lifestyle, start by taking a small step. Take a couple of weeks to pay attention to the glycemic index of the foods that you are eating. Plan your meals around foods that have a low glycemic load.

Let me give you a list of foods that are low on the glycemic index, and then I will give you a list of foods that are high up on the list. And then, you can make decisions about your meal plan for the next week or even for just the next few days.

Foods That Are <u>Low</u> on the Glycemic Index According to Healthline.Com (Coyle, 2017)

- Bread: whole grain, multigrain, rye, and sourdough varieties

- Breakfast cereals: rolled oats, Bircher muesli, and all bran

- Fruit: apples, strawberries, apricots, peaches, plums, pears, and kiwi

- Vegetables: carrots, broccoli, cauliflower, celery, tomatoes, and zucchini

- Starchy vegetables: Charisma and Nicola potato varieties, sweet potatoes, corn, and yams

- Legumes: lentils, chickpeas, baked beans, butter beans, and kidney beans

- Pasta and noodles: soba noodles, vermicelli noodles, and rice noodles

- Rice: Basmati, Doongara, long-grain, and brown rice

- Grains: quinoa, barley, pearl couscous, buckwheat, freekeh, and semolina

- Dairy: milk, cheese, yogurt, custard, soy milk, and almond milk

Food Without a GI Value

- Meat: beef, chicken, pork, lamb, and eggs
- Fish and seafood: salmon, trout, tuna, sardines, and prawns
- Nuts: almonds, cashews, pistachios, walnuts, and macadamia nuts
- Fats and oils: olive oil, rice bran oil, butter, and margarine
- Herbs and spices: salt, pepper, garlic, basil, and dill

Remember that the goal here is just to have foods that are low to moderate on the Glycemic Index. Some of the items on this list would not be included in some low carb diets that completely restrict the consumption of carbohydrates. We will discuss these diets in Chapter Eight.

Foods to Avoid Because They Are High on the Glycemic Index (Coyle, 2017)

- Bread: white bread, French baguettes, bagels, and any bread made with refined flour such as Turkish or Lebanese breads

- Breakfast cereals: instant oats, Rice Krispies, Corn Flakes, Cocoa Krispies, and Fruit Loops

- Starchy vegetables: potatoes (Desiree and Red Pontiac potatoes) and instant mashed potatoes

- Pasta and noodles: corn pasta and instant noodles

- Rice: Jasmine, Arborio (risotto Calrose), and medium grain white rice

- Dairy replacements: rice milk and oat milk

- Fruit: watermelon

- Savory snacks: rice crackers, corn tins, rice cakes, pretzels, corn chips, and potato chips

- Cakes and biscuits: scones, doughnuts, cupcakes, cookies, and waffles

- Candies: jellybeans, chocolate bars, and lollipops

Remember that it is the small steps that you take over time that help you to get to the goals that you want to achieve. By paying attention to the glycemic index and glycemic load, you will enjoy a smoother transition to a healthy eating plan or diet.

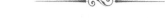

CHAPTER SUMMARY

- PCOS and insulin sensitivity are linked together.
- The glycemic index and glycemic load are important to know.
- Healthy eating can reverse the effects of insulin sensitivity.

In the next chapter, you will learn about the Anti-Inflammatory Diet.

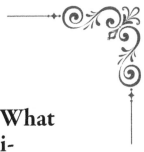

Chapter Six: What Is an Anti-inflammatory Diet and Do I Need It?

Inflammation and PCOS

One of the latest discoveries about PCOS is that it is linked to inflammatory responses in the body. To understand what inflammation means to the body, think about bruises and how the body swells up around that bruise. The swelling or inflammation happens because the body is trying to protect the injured area. Specifically, inflammation is found when the body is protecting you from harmful bacteria, viruses, and injury. Inflammation is good when it is protecting you, but sometimes inflammation can be a sign that your body is attacking healthy cells and organs (Morris, 2011).

Why does the medical community think that inflammation and PCOS go together? Inflammation doesn't just happen in a vacuum. When inflammation is present in the body, there are certain signs in the body like elevated levels of a C-reactive protein called CRP. Women with PCOS are found to have elevated levels of this protein.

Also present when there is an inflammation in your body is oxidative stress. This kind of stress in your body happens when there are "free radicals that overwhelm your body's defenses against harmful effects" (Morris, 2011). Also present in the body when there is inflammation are inflammatory cytokines and white blood cells (lymphocytes and monocytes) (Morris, 2011).

When women with PCOS are tested, these markers are found in their system. Moreover, elevated CRP is found in people with diabetes, insulin resistance, and heart disease. Women with PCOS sometimes have these conditions. Consequently, some doctors believe that inflammation might be the root cause of PCOS.

As discussed in earlier chapters, women with PCOS have excess androgens. These excess androgens cause higher insulin levels and those levels "contribute to weight gain which causes more inflammation" (Grassi, 2018).

The Mediterian Diet and Symptoms of PCOS and Inflammation

If a woman with PCOS changes her diet, she can relieve some of the symptoms of PCOS and inflammation. In a study published by the *North American Journal of Medical Sciences*, researchers discovered that diet can improve inflammatory disease and PCOS in women.

This study followed women with PCOS for three months. Each woman was required to follow a Mediterranean style anti-inflammatory diet for three months. In particular, the study investigated the effects of the diet, known for its anti-inflammatory properties, on overweight and obese women with PCOS.

The Mediterranean style diet follows a 25% protein, 25% fat, and 50% carbohydrate formula and focuses on anti-inflammatory foods such as fish, legumes, nuts, olive oil, herbs spices, and green tea. The women followed this diet, and in the end, they lost 7% of their body weight and their cholesterol, blood pressure, and inflammatory markers improved. A whopping 63% of the women got their menstrual cycles back and 12% got pregnant. Subsequently, if you have PCOS, you might want to follow a diet with anti-inflammatory properties.

The Anti-inflammatory Diet

Anti-inflammatory diets are created to be low calorie, low-fat, low saturated fat, and moderate to high fiber. This diet also suggests what to eat and how to eat it. For example, you will be eating a diet that is half carbohydrates so you should evenly space out carbs during the day. Moreover, when you serve your plate, fill one half of the plate with vegetables and also eat a variety of fruits.

Other foods that you are encouraged to eat are beans and legumes, several times a week, and foods rich in omega-3, such as salmon, tuna, and trout, at least two times a week. It is also recommended that the 25% of fat that you need to consume comes from unsaturated sources of fat that can be found in flaxseeds, olive oil, and nuts. The anti-inflammatory diet also encourages you to drink green tea daily and have red meat only twice a month (Grassi, 2018).

Herbs and spices are also known to fight inflammation. Here are some examples of special herbs and spices and what they do in the fight to prevent inflammation.

- Cayenne pepper helps to fight cancer and cleans out the arteries.

- Cumin helps flush toxins from the body and prevents cancer.

- Garlic is anti-inflammatory. It also has antiviral and antibacterial properties.

- Ginger helps with inflammation that causes joint pain.

- Turmeric relieves arthritis, tendonitis, and some autoimmune disorders (Morris, 2011).

Foods that increase inflammation are: trans fats, refined sugars, and artificial foods. Some examples of these foods are cookies, doughnuts, pastries, white bread, prepared salad dressings and condiments, sugary cereals, sodas, French fries, margarine, potatoes, corn chips, fried foods, and anything made with bleached or enriched flour.

The Inflammation Index

In 2009, researchers at the University of South Carolina and the University of Massachusetts put together an inflammation index. They studied more than 60 years of reports, studies, and articles on "foods and how their individual compounds affected the body" (Morris, 2011). The researchers were able to score foods by determining whether they were anti-inflammatory or inflammatory.

The researchers gave each food a rating called the inflammation factor (IF). Foods that are anti-inflammatory have positive ratings and foods with inflammatory qualities have negative ratings. Researchers set a target rating of 50 to identify how well you are following the anti-inflammatory diet. For example, you can still eat foods with a negative inflammatory rating, but you have to balance it out with a positive number. For example, if you drink a soda with a negative number of -50, you can balance it out by eating something with a greater positive rating that will absorb the negative number.

Good Fats and the Anti-inflammatory Diet

Good fats such as unsaturated fats, both monounsaturated and polyunsaturated, are important to the anti-inflammatory diet. Good fats help keep inflammation in your body from happening. Stay away from trans fats, as they are not part of the anti-inflammatory diet. Saturated fats are divided by good saturated fats and not so good fats. Itis recommended that in a 2,000 a day calorie diet, only 140 calories should be from saturated fat (Morris, 2011).

Examples of sources of monounsaturated fats are avocado, olive oil, olives, almonds, pecans, sunflower oil, sesame oil, grapeseed oil, and oatmeal. Examples of sources of polyunsaturated fats are salmon, trout, sardines, soybeans, walnuts, flaxseeds, and wheat germ. An example of a good saturated fat is coconut oil.

Trans fats are the fats that you must stay away from. Foods that have trans fats are biscuits, cakes, pastries, doughnuts, shortening, and microwave popcorn.

The Anti-Inflammatory Diet and Carbohydrates

Unlike the keto diet and other low carb diets, the anti-inflammatory diet recommends that 50% of your diet should be carbohydrates. Can you believe this? The anti-inflammatory diet wants you to get your energy not from fat but from carbohydrates. Of course, this diet distinguishes some carbs to be good and other carbs to be not so good for you.

The main function of carbohydrates is to provide energy for your muscles and central nervous system; prevent protein from being used as energy; enable fatty acid breakdown for fats and energy; and provide the body with sources of fiber (Morris, 2011).

The inflammation diet takes into consideration that there are simple carbs and complex carbs. The simple carbs are broken down and absorbed quickly in your system, and the complex carbs take longer to break down.

Did you know that fiber is considered a carb? It's considered to be so complex, it can't be broken down by the body, and consequently, goes through the body without being digested. As it passes through the body, it keeps our bowels healthy and helps us to control our blood sugar levels. There are two types of fiber, soluble fiber, and insoluble fiber.

The tricky thing about carbohydrates is that in certain combinations, they can raise our blood sugar. High blood sugar causes inflammation. On the anti-inflammatory diet, instead of not eating carbs, you make sure to eat complex carbs to reduce inflammation.

In an anti-inflammatory diet you will find that processed foods are not allowed. When a food is processed and becomes refined, it not only loses fiber but also vitamins, minerals, and other important nutrients.

Proteins and the Anti-Inflammatory Diet

Proteins are important to an anti-inflammatory diet because humans need amino acids to build muscles. Out of the 22 amino acids required to make protein, our body only makes 13. So, we need to find foods that can provide us with the amino acids that we need.

Protein is necessary because it helps us repair damaged tissues, build muscles, and it feeds our blood. Insulin is one example of a protein in our body. Proteins are also important to our immune system, and antibodies are proteins. The C-reactive protein (CPR) that we mentioned at the beginning of this chapter gets sent out by the body to signal illness or injury. When the levels of CPR are high, it indicates that there is inflammation in your body.

Foods That Are Good for You

The Mediterranean diet is a good example of an anti-inflammatory diet but there are also foods that you can eat on a regular basis to help reduce the inflammation in your body.

Salmon

A major source of protein, salmon is an essential ingredient to any anti-inflammatory diet. Rich in omega-3 fatty acids, salmon helps reduce the risk of heart and cardiovascular disease, strokes, and heart arrhythmias. But the most important benefit that salmon can bring to a diet is that it really makes you feel full. Also, it helps your body respond to insulin for better blood sugar control. Try to fit salmon into your diet at least two to three times a week.

Flaxseeds

A tiny brown seed from the Linum usitatissimum plant, flaxseed has been around for centuries. Flaxseeds have a high amount of omega-3 fatty acids and help fight inflammation in the body. Flaxseeds also have phytoestrogens that act as selective estrogen response modifiers (SERM) in the same way as the breast cancer drug Tamoxifen. SERMS boost estrogen when it is low in the body, and when estrogen is high, SERMS can reduce estrogen levels.

Flaxseeds are also high in manganese, folate, copper, phosphorus, and vitamin B6.

Blueberries

High in antioxidants, blueberries protect cells from inflammation and oxidative stress. Blueberries also have fiber, manganese, and vitamins C, E and K.

Almonds

Natural almonds have monounsaturated fat, protein, and potassium. They promote heart health. They also have vitamin E, an antioxidant that prevents heart attacks. The most important thing that almonds do for women with PCOS is they help slow down the rise in insulin and blood sugar. Almonds are known to help fight insulin resistance.

Mushrooms

A popular food that has many benefits, mushrooms contain considerable amounts of antioxidants, phytonutrients and polysaccharides, which regulate the immune system. Mushrooms can help you regulate your blood sugar, so they are a big help in your fight against insulin resistance. Mushrooms are also known to help increase ovulation in women with PCOS.

Broccoli

A superfood that his high in dietary fiber, broccoli helps to keep your intestines clean and helps with insulin resistance. Broccoli contain vitamins C and D, calcium, iron folate, and phytonutrients.

Quinoa

A whole grain that is a complete protein, quinoa is gluten-free and is high in magnesium and riboflavin. Quinoa helps with inflammation in blood vessels. Quinoa also helps with insulin resistance and is high in manganese, magnesium, iron, tryptophan copper, and phosphorus. Substituting quinoa for carbohydrates at least three to five times a week can really be beneficial to you in many ways.

Brussel Sprouts

A hearty cruciferous vegetable, brussels sprouts are high in antioxidants and omega-3s. Brussel sprouts are also known to be an immense help in detoxification. High in fiber that can help with insulin resistance, brussels sprouts contain vitamins K,C,A, B6, B1, B2 and E, folate, manganese, potassium, tryptophan, iron, phosphorus, magnesium, copper, and calcium.

Onions

Full of anti-inflammatory benefits, onions aid in detoxification and they boost immune function. Important to women with PCOS, onions help to improve sugar control and improve insulin resistance. Onions are high in chromium, vitamins C and B6, manganese, molybdenum, tryptophan, folate, potassium, phosphorus, and copper.

Anti-Inflammatory Supplements and Herbs

It is important to a woman with PCOS that she reduce inflammation in her body. Here are some supplements, natural herbs, and enzymes that will help fight inflammation. As always, consult a specialist who is remarkably familiar with these herbs and enzymes, and the treatment of PCOS and inflammation.

Omega-3 Fatty Acids

There are two essential fatty acids: eicosapentaenoic acid (EPA) and docosahexaenoic acid (DHA) that come from fish and vegetarian sources. It is important to have these present in our system to fight inflammation. These essential fatty acids are considered anti-inflammatory superstars (Morris, 2011).

Foods that have these omega-3 fatty acids are fish (salmon and sardines), fish oils, flax, and chia seeds. Flax and chia seeds have alpha linolenic acid (ALA) that gets converted into EPA. It is especially important to choose high quality supplements.

Ginger

The root of the ginger plant has multiple anti-inflammatory benefits. It decreases inflammation, pain, and risk of heart and cardiovascular disease. It is also antibacterial and antifungal.

Turmeric/Curcumin

The root of the Indian Curcuma longa plant contains an extract called curcumin and has multiple anti-inflammatory benefits. Curcumin has a bright orange color and acts in the same way as ibuprofen.

NAC (N-Acetyl Cysteine)

NAC (N-Acetyl Cysteine) is a derivative of amino acids. It acts as an antioxidant and stops inflammation. It also reduces free-radical damage.

Bromelain

An enzyme derived from pineapple, bromelain decreases the inflammatory response of the immune system and works as an antioxidant to increase reactive oxygen species (ROS) that cleans up the "mess" made by inflammation.

Boswellia

Indian frankincense Boswellia has boswellic acid and alpha and beta boswellic acid that has anti-inflammatory properties.

Vitamin D

A fat-soluble vitamin that boosts the immune system and reduces the risks of bone fractures.

Vitamin C

Ascorbic acid or vitamin C decreases inflammation by being a potent antioxidant. Vitamin C decreases the C-reactive protein that is elevated when your body is inflamed. Sources for vitamin C are broccoli, papaya, bell peppers, oranges, cantaloupes, kiwis, cauliflower, brussels sprouts, and strawberries.

Papain

An enzyme derived from papaya, it helps reduce inflammation by breaking down harmful substances in the body.

Coenzyme Q10

A vitamin like substance, Coenzyme Q10 supplies energy to all cells of the body. It is an antioxidant and helps stabilize cell membranes.

Making the Difference

Anti-inflammatory food and supplements can really make a difference in healthy eating. Following an anti-inflammatory diet can go a long way in healing your body from PCOS. A good start for beginning an anti-inflammatory diet is to include the foods that are mentioned in this chapter. Instead of concentrating on what you need to take out of your diet, adding these anti-inflammatory foods and supplements can really boost your health.

So often, diets are hard to follow because you must remove foods that you love from your daily meals. Instead, make small changes like adding blueberries to a low-fat pudding or chopping up a half cup of onions and throwing them into your favorite casserole. It's just that easy to help yourself heal from the damage that inflammation causes in your system.

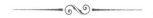

CHAPTER SUMMARY

- In an anti-inflammatory diet, 50% of your diet is made up of carbohydrates.

- High blood sugar causes inflammation.

- There are foods and supplements that can help reduce inflammation.

In the next chapter, you will learn about diet breaks.

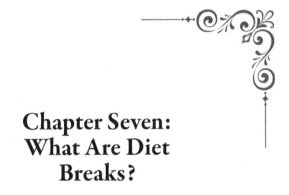

Chapter Seven:
What Are Diet
Breaks?

The following chapter was inspired by the book _The Guide to Flexible Dieting_, by Lyle MacDonald as discussed by Andy Morgan at rippedbody.com/diet-break/.

When you are looking to make a lifestyle change for your health, you need to do something that is do-able. You can't choose to do something so difficult that you break down and feel like a failure. If you go to this extreme, you won't get anything done. If you choose to do something that is just a little bit out of your comfort zone, chances are that you are going to have success and even be willing to go a step further in your quest for change.

In the earlier chapters, we established that insulin resistance is one of the most serious symptoms of PCOS. One of the ways to reduce insulin resistance is to eat a healthier diet that will result in weight loss. The longer you wait to start a healthy diet, the more the symptoms of PCOS will set in. To this end, we will discuss several different diets, but I found something in my research that I would like to share with you: diet breaks.

What Is a Diet Break?

A diet break is a planned break from your diet. It can last for a day to two weeks. During this break, you simply eat more calories than what you eat when you are on the diet. This break means that you take a vacation from following your diet and you "free-style" it for a day or even a week. When you vacation, you relax from your usual routine and prepare yourself for what is ahead. Diets can be stressful with all the different demands that are made on you.

When you are on a diet, you must follow a regime and a routine that supports your weight loss. If you "cheat" and eat more, for example, you have defeated and sometimes even wiped out all the work you did before. How does a diet break different than a cheat day? Or, are they the same? Well, let's face it, we are not machines. There are going to be meals or even whole days that we cheat. It's just human nature. If your diet leaves you hungry, perhaps on a certain day you just don't have the mental ability to not think about being hungry. You've had that capacity, for let's say three weeks, but at the start of your fourth week, your attitude changes and you "cheat."

Knowing that this is in our nature, we can stay ahead of the game if we plan for that day or days that we are going to drop out of our regimen and routines.

What Does a Diet Break Look Like?

An example of a diet break is a scheduled 7-14 day where you purposefully increase calorie intake and stop minding all the restrictions that are put in place by your diet. On a diet, you can have a day off like on your birthday or for the holidays. A diet break is different than a day off because you will have a plan for this break. You are not going to just stuff your face.

You are taking a semi-disciplined break. Since you are increasing your calories, you will gain weight. However, according to Andy Morgan, you are not going to gain a lot of fat.

During this break, you are going to eat until you are full and reach for that second or third helping that you usually deny yourself. How can this result in not gaining any fat?

Morgan explains that it takes a 3,500-calorie surplus to gain 1lb of fat. His theory is that you won't overeat as much as you think you are going to, since you've been on a diet and controlling the amount of food that you eat. It's kind of like if you are used to eating on saucer and you move up to a salad plate, your brain interprets that as a lot of food. You won't jump to eating a platter's worth of food. Morgan believes that you won't eat more than 1,000 calories over what you usually eat. Perhaps you have been on your diet long enough that you have already been making lifestyle choices that will cancel out the unhealthy habits that you had before. Morgan even has a theory that for every 1 gram of carb intake, it brings along 3-4 grams of water with it. This can be a weight gain of water and not fat.

How Does a Diet Break Help?

Taking a diet break helps the body recover from any major changes that it has been making during your diet. In essence, you are giving your body time to catch up on the changes that have been happening since you've been eating less, or in the case of a diet like the keto diet, eating differently. Psychologically, everyone needs a vacation from challenging work.

You can either go on a full diet break or be just a little different than your usual diet days and keep some control. During a full break, you will be eating until you are no longer hungry, as discussed before. You will stop counting your macronutrients, but you will keep your regular mealtimes. You will keep doing your physical regimen, as in not stopping from those long walks or runs you've been taking. All you will be doing is eating more.

If you don't want the freedom to eat until you are full, a more controlled diet break is something you will feel more comfortable doing. For example, when you are on the keto diet, you stay with the keto formula of 75% fat, 20% protein, and 5% carbs. On the controlled break, you might just count calories instead of having to stick to that formula.

Overall, during the diet break, you will raise your calories by 500 every day or to a level where you will maintain but not gain weight. You won't work so hard on hitting your macronutrient totals, but instead do something simple like maintaining a calorie intake. You will also cut in half the type of exercise you do to burn calories, and instead do something like yoga or just stretching. The amount of days that you are going to take off will be anywhere from 10-14 days. The difference here is that you don't indulge in a whole lot of unhealthy foods. You keep eating healthy, you just eat a little bit more of the healthy stuff. Plus, you stay active.

The Study That Proves Everything

There is a study that supports Lyle McDonald's theory of diet breaks. The study is called *Prescribed "Breaks" as a Means to Disrupt Weight Control Efforts* by Rena R. Wing and Robert W. Jeffery (2002).

In this study, Wing and Jeffery found that diet breaks are not detrimental to a person's weight loss goals. Here is a description of their study and what they learned:

When a person is dieting, can they take a break and not gain weight? For example, some people go off their diet during birthdays and holidays. Is it possible that these people will not gain weight? In this study, 142 people followed a 14-week diet program, with 14 weekly lessons. One group, the "LB" group, took a 6-week break after lesson 7 and the "SB" group took 2-week breaks after lessons 3, 6, and 9. During the breaks, the participants were asked to stop their diets. The participants did stop their diet, but they kept up their weight loss activities like exercise. In the end, the study proved that there were no adverse effects to taking breaks.

A key takeaway here is that it is hard for people who diet to stick to their diets for a continuous amount of time. Usually, at six months, the dieter gives up and experiences weight gain. But what if you were able to adjust the way you think and take breaks to help you keep dieting in the long term? The researchers felt that the reasons dieters quit is because they have problems with "psychological and behavioral adjustment to the process of weight loss" (Wing & Jeffery, 2002) regardless of physiological reasons. In other words, quitting your diet is a mind thing and not a body thing.

The researchers hoped that during this study, they could learn more about why a person quits a diet. Dieters seem to get a momentum for dieting, and they are rewarded with consistent weight loss. Then, something happens, and their momentum is broken, and they begin to gain weight again. Is it possible that you could take assigned breaks and not gain weight and then get back to dieting after the break? Most importantly, could this happen without gaining any additional weight?

In this study, the 142 participants all took part in group meetings. These meetings consisted of a weigh-in, discussion, and lesson focused on diet, exercise and behavioral strategies. Participants were all on a diet of 1000-1500 calories. Each participant was given a list of 13 high fat foods that they couldn't eat, and they took part in 150 minutes of activity per week. Each participant wrote down information about their diet and exercise programs and they weighed themselves daily. Plus, during the meetings the participants were given a questionnaire to complete about how often over the previous week they had eaten one of the 13 high fat foods that they were told to avoid, the number of days that they weighed themselves, the number of days that they recorded their diet and exercise, and the number of minutes they spent walking over that past week.

The dieters were informed that the breaks were given to them so that they could learn how to recover from diet breaks. They didn't attend group meetings during their breaks, and they were told not to check their behavior or weight during the weeks that they were off. The participants were told that they could go back to the eating and exercise routines they had before they started the study. There were no interventions when the participants came back, other than the prevention lessons that they received at their weekly meetings. After the participants finished the program, they were encouraged to keep up the diet and exercise programs they had learned while being part of the study.

Here is a graph that illustrates the progress of the participants during the study:

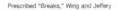

Prescribed "Breaks," Wing and Jeffery

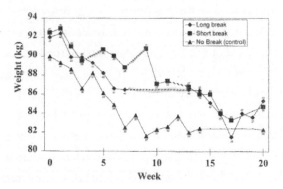

Table 1 Source: **"Prescribed "Breaks" as a Means to Disrupt Weight Control Efforts"** by Rena R. Wing and Robert W. Jeffery, July 29, 2002.

Table 1 illustrates the "weight of participants in the no break (control) group, the LB and SB, over the course of the initial 20 weeks of the study. Periods where the participants were instructed to take a "break" from the program are indicated by dashed lines. Number of participants available at each session is indicated on the graph" (Wing & Jeffery, 2002).

Although the participants gained insignificant amounts of weight or stayed the same during the breaks, there wasn't a significant difference between either the control group or the groups that took the break.

The findings of the study

The study found that the participants were able to take the long or short breaks without "subsequent adverse effects on continued adherence to the program goals or overall weight loss" (Wing & Jeffery, 2002), proving that taking breaks are not bad for dieters. According to the information on the questionnaire that the participants filled out, they took breaks from weighing themselves and they ate the restricted food items, but they did not stop their activity. This gave the researchers the idea that the participants enjoyed the activity part of the study, so much so, that they did not stop during the breaks.

The researchers felt that the most important question of their study was: Why didn't the breaks disrupt the adherence to the diet or the participants' weight loss? The researchers noted that the breaks didn't disrupt the dieters because they were told to take the breaks, as opposed to when dieters stop dieting on their own due to negative thoughts or circumstances.

This study was important because it proved that dieters can take breaks and not gain a lot of weight or stop a diet forever. The participants in the program were able to get right back to the diet after the breaks. Plus, the dieters stayed active, even though they weren't on program. This is good news because so often dieters take breaks on holidays and birthdays. This study proves that it is possible to take breaks and then go back to your diet without any negative outcomes. Furthermore, taking diet breaks might just be good practice for people who want to lose weight.

A key point of the diet break study is that the participants continued to exercise while they were on break. This highlights the importance of exercising while you are trying to lose weight. Perhaps, if the study participants had not exercised, they would have gained weight.

I know it's hard to stay on a diet. You start out strong, but then after a few weeks, your motivation fizzles away. This has happened to me more than a few times. First, I get excited about a diet plan, so I rush out and buy two weeks worth of food that is on the meal plan. Then, after those two weeks, I repeat the meal plan and finish a month of dieting. Yet, at the beginning of the next month, I find myself bored of the diet, and I fall off the wagon. If this cycle sounds familiar, diet breaks might be just what you need to get back on track.

I love the idea of taking a break between diet weeks. I know I could do that. I wouldn't even mind exercising. In my experience, it's easier to keep exercise interesting. You could try a new class or change up the machines you use like swapping the treadmill for an exercise bike.

Overall, it is good to know that taking breaks from your diet might not be a big deal if you continue to exercise. Will you give this a try? Personally, I think diet breaks might be the best invention since Diet Coke!

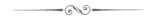

CHAPTER SUMMARY

- A diet break is a planned break from a diet.

- On a diet break, you eat more than you planned to eat. This is called "free-styling" it.

- When you are on a diet break, continue to exercise to reduce your chances of gaining weight.

In the next chapter, you will learn about the keto diet.

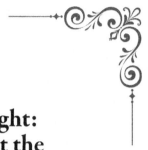

Chapter Eight: What About the Keto Diet for PCOS?

A common trait among most women who have PCOS is being overweight due to insulin resistance. In this chapter, we are going to examine the keto diet and analyze the pros and cons of being on the keto diet and reversing insulin resistance. Of all the low carb diets, the ketogenic diet is the biggest challenge. Why? Well, for it to work, you must get into a state of ketosis. And, to get into this state, you have to deprive the body of enough carbohydrates to make glucose. When your body isn't getting its energy from carbs, it will be forced to go into fat reserves and burn fat for fuel. As this process happens, your body creates acids that are called ketones. By measuring these ketones, you can determine whether or not your body has reached ketosis.

A Century of the Ketogenic Diet

The ketogenic diet was conceived almost a hundred years ago and has been successful for children who suffer from epilepsy. The keto diet was so successful, that many children and adults who followed this diet, never had another seizure again. Along the way, someone noticed that going into ketosis helped people lose weight, and the keto diet craze was started. I remember in the 1970's my hard-working, cynical father tried the keto diet and lost weight. I didn't know exactly what the keto diet was when I was a child, but I knew that you had to pee on a strip to know whether it was working or not.

Getting to Ketosis and Staying There

That's the trouble with the keto diet, you must stay in ketosis for it to work. And, to get into ketosis, you all but have to eliminate carbohydrates. In fact, you must follow the keto diet formula of 75% fat, 20% protein, and 5% carbohydrates. How do you do something like that? Well, you've got to learn which micronutrients to have in your diet so that you can achieve ketosis, and this is a lot harder than you might think. First, every individual is different when it comes to exactly how many grams of fat, protein, and carbs it takes to achieve the keto formula. There is no one-size-fits-all formula for everybody. It's a lot of trial and error with the diet and a lot of testing (urine, blood, or breath) to know if you've reached ketosis.

The keto formula, 75-20-5, doesn't tell you how much to eat. You figure that out using a keto calculator or a fancy formula to determine first, how many calories you need to eat, or not eat, to lose weight. Once you've got that number, then you can figure out the grams of fat, protein, and carbs you need. These are called macronutrients. I'm not saying that you can't follow a meal plan written out in a keto diet book to find success. It's pretty much just hit or miss. But with a keto-calculator, you can figure out the exact amounts of macronutrients that you are going to need.

Let's say you get all the macronutrients squared away and now you are on your way to losing weight on the keto diet. When you are in the process of getting into ketosis, you are going to experience the keto flu. This is the result of going cold turkey on carbohydrates. The keto flu can be mild and only last a couple of days, or it can be severe and last for weeks, or in extreme cases, months. People who have gone through this really know the importance of staying on the diet and keeping that state of ketosis going because who wants to go through the keto flu twice?

While you are in ketosis, you must drink a lot of water because the process of burning fat really gets rid of the water in your body, so you need to replace it. Also, by cutting a majority of carbs from your diet, you will have to compensate by taking supplements of vitamins and minerals.

Keto Diet and Fun

It can be fun being on the keto diet, especially once you get over the flu. Why? Well you get to eat your weight in bacon (well, almost) and you get to enjoy good, healthy fat again without feeling guilty. There are even "fat bombs" that are highly concentrated, good fat snacks that help you hit that 75% sweet spot. I've seen recipes for chocolate chip and carrot cake fat bombs that really look amazing. When I tried the Atkins diet (a form of the keto diet) back in the early 2000s, I didn't have the chance to try fat bombs, but I did enjoy eating a lot of bratwurst and pork rinds. I know a lot more about the keto diet now, and looking back, I don't think I ever really stayed in a state of ketosis. It was kind of hit or miss. However, I did learn to cut back on carbs and concentrate on protein. In fact, that was the way I learned to make eating protein my main goal.

I lost thirty pounds and the Atkins diet changed the way I felt about carbs. To this day, I no longer have cereal for breakfast, and I stay away from sugar. Two good things that have served me well.

Although I've made an argument for why the keto diet is hard to follow (the personalized macronutrients), there is an argument to be made that with a good keto calculator app and the sheer will of staying away from sugar and processed foods, the keto diet can be a good system for following a low carb diet. One of the greatest characteristics of the keto diet is the fact that because of all the good fat and protein that you are eating, you stay full longer. You don't get that starving feeling or gnawing hunger from eating too many carbs. We all know the drill – your carbo load and thirty minutes later, you are back for more carbs. Since you stay feeling full, you are more likely to stay on the diet. And, the longer you stay on this diet, the more weight you are going to lose.

So, what does this mean for women like you who are suffering from PCOS?

I am going to tell you about two studies that were done where women with PCOS followed the keto diet and found success.

Two Studies of the Ketogenic Diet
A Ketogenic Diet May Restore Fertility in Women With Polycystic Ovary Syndrome: A Case Series

In this study, four women with confirmed cases of PCOS followed the keto diet for six months. They went to the study site once a month for a check-up and to be assessed for weight loss, menstrual regularity, and ovulation.

Here are some key facts about PCOS that the researchers focused on: PCOS is the most common reason for infertility in women. This type of infertility happens when you don't have regular periods throughout the year. When you don't have a period, it is likely that you have not ovulated.

The majority of women with PCOS are obese (80%) and they have insulin resistance. There are women who have PCOS who are not obsese. However, these women have insulin resistance. Perhaps not as severe as a woman who is obese. Specifically, the woman who is obese has had insulin resistance longer - that is why she is obese. (Insulin resistance has brought about more insulin in her system which has slowed her metabolic rate.)

Insulin resistance is the main "disturbance" in women with PCOS. It makes sense that the researchers wanted their subjects to have insulin resistance, because this type of disturbance is the precursor to other symptoms like excess androgens.

Increased insulin increases androgen levels. As discussed in Chapter Four, when there is too much insulin being released into your bloodstream, your ovaries begin to secrete more androgens.

Patients with insulin resistance are often resistant to ovulation induction; specifically, these women do not respond to the infertility medication that they are given.

The Results of the Study

When the women restricted their carb intake and went into ketosis, signs and symptoms of insulin resistance either improved or went away completely. The women began to ovulate regularly, and in doing so, they increased their chances of fertility.

The Effects of a Low-Carbohydrate, Ketogenic Diet on the Polycystic Ovary Syndrome: A Pilot Study

This study was a lot like the first one. Eleven women were recruited to limit their carb intake to 20 grams or less for 24 weeks. Every two weeks, the patients checked in. In the end, only five women were able to finish the study. Two of those women became pregnant, even though they had infertility problems before the study.

What We Can Learn From These Studies

When the women in the study followed a low-carb, ketogenic diet, they lost a significant amount of weight and had improvements in their free testosterone LH/FSH ratio and fasting insulin.

Does this mean that everyone who has PCOS and insulin resistance should go on the keto diet? Well, three major advantages to the keto diet is that after you get the knack of counting your macronutrients, it is easy to follow, you aren't as hungry, and it is good for your insulin. In the second study, out of the 11 women that were recruited, only five managed to finish the study. Yet, remember that out of those five, two became pregnant!

Further Study

Both studies say that further examination of the keto diet and women with PCOS is needed. The keto diet is a controversial diet. One argument is that practically cutting out carbs is not good for you. Specifically, if you eat very few carbs, you are missing out on some of the vitamins and minerals that we receive from carbohydrates. Of course, everyone can benefit from staying away from processed foods and refined sugar. No one is going to argue this point. Yet, when you are on the keto diet, you can't have bananas, oranges, or apples. With this in mind, let's take a closer look at the requirements of the keto diet.

The Requirements of the Keto Diet

When you go "keto" it is important to follow the keto diet formula which is 75% fat, 20% protein, and 5% carbohydrates. The percentages of these macronutrients are very important because this is what is going to put your body into ketosis and get it burning stored fat for energy.

In order to achieve 75% fat, you need to eat foods with healthy fats. Yes, it is true that you get to eat a lot of bacon, but you also eat foods like cheese and avocados that have a lot of good fat. In order to achieve the 20% protein, it is smart to eat foods like salmon and and quinoa to get the maximum in healthy protein. However, the trick is going to be that you don't eat a lot of carbs. The biggest misunderstanding of the keto diet is that you don't have any carbs at all. This is not necessarily true. It is very important to get the vitamins and minerals that are in foods like blueberries and tomatoes. Carbs give you energy, and although eating more protein is going to help you stay full longer, you will still crave carbs to get you through that energy crunch.

Another important point is that each person has their own unique calorie needs and these unique needs – specifically your total calorie number like 2,000 – will determine the grams of fat, protein and carbohydrates that make up the percentages of your macronutrients.

There are formulas to help you find these "numbers" but the easiest thing to do is download keto calculators that can easily calculate what your "numbers" are going to be. Your "numbers" are going to change as you lose weight, and they also change when you exercise. You are allowed to carbo load to a point when you are going to be expending a lot of energy like when you exercise. Using a keto calculator to work out your "numbers" for you when you exercise will be a big help.

Once you get into ketosis, you are going to want to stay there. This is the hardest part of the keto diet – and that's sticking to the food plan so that you continue to burn fat. However, a plus with the keto diet is that you are most likely not going to feel hungry. Eating foods that are high in good fats and protein makes you feel more satiated or full. Not starving on your diet, goes a long way in keeping you on it.

Below are foods that you can incorporate into your meal plan to get you into ketosis.

Keto-Friendly Foods

- Seafood

- Low carb vegetables

- Low sugar fruits like tomatoes, avocado, blackberries, raspberries, blueberries, strawberries, coconut, lemons, and limes

- Dairy like cheese, cottage cheese, plain Greek yogurt, cream, butter (notice milk is missing)

- Avocados

- Meat and poultry

- Eggs

● Nuts like macadamia nuts, flaxseed, brazil nuts, chia seeds, walnuts, pecans, hemp seeds, hazelnuts, sesame seeds, pumping seeds, and almonds (notice that peanuts are missing because they are considered a legume)

● Oils like extra-virgin olive oil, coconut oil, avocado oil, nut oils, coconut butter, MCT oil (notice vegetable, canola and peanut oil are not included)

● Dark chocolate (at least 70% cacao)

● Bread made with amaranth, almond, and other flours that do not come from wheat

Foods That Are Not Keto Friendly

When you go on a keto diet, you are staying away from anything that is high in carbohydrates. This requirement has you staying away from processed foods and refined sugar. Mainly, you should avoid eating foods that get quickly turned into glucose. Getting into ketosis will require you to give your body such a low supply of glucose, it has to turn to your liver to release its energy sources i.e. glycogen.

Complex carbohydrates take longer to digest, so there is less glucose in your bloodstream when you eat these types of carbohydrates. You may think that breads made with wheat flour or legumes like peanuts, chick peas or kidney beans might be keto friendly because they have fiber and are considered a complex carbohydrate. The problem with this type of food is that they are high in carbs.

You will have to rethink foods like hummus or peanut butter because of their carb counts. Just one tablespoon of chickpeas has 8 grams of carbs. This doesn't sound bad, but when you mash it up into hummus, you are eating concentrated chickpeas with a carb count of 35 grams in one cup of hummus. Of course, you might only eat half a cup and that would be 17.5 grams of carbohydrates. Some people still include hummus in their keto diet because they add a lot of olive oil as a healthy fat. Again, your personal macronutrient counts will be important here. If you are very active and burn a lot of energy from exercise or exertion at work, 17.5 grams might fit into your meal plan. Use a keto-calculator to find your macros before you have that half cup of hummus.

Other foods that are not keto-friendly are milk and cereals like oatmeal and cream of wheat. When you can't have foods that are not keto-friendly, you have to get to know the things that you can have. For example, pancakes made with regular white flour is not keto-friendly. Yet, if you made pancakes out of almond or amaranth flour, you would be able to have pancakes. The same goes for things like pudding. I am a big fan of tapioca, but it has a lot of carbs. I learned that you can use chia seeds, soak them in milk and you have a pudding that is a lot like tapioca.

It's important to find a good keto diet cookbook so that you can learn about foods that you can substitute for the foods that are not keto-friendly. Rest assured, keto is not about what you can't have but what you **can** have.

Does the Keto Diet Deprive you of Vitamins and Minerals?

It's a toss up as to whether you are deprived of essential vitamins and minerals if you are on a keto diet. This factor depends a lot on what your food choices are going to be. For example, you might go without eating peanuts, but you could eat macadamia nuts or pecans instead. Do peanuts bring to the table anything that macadamias or pecans don't?

Do you really miss anything by going without processed food? Did anyone ever die from not eating out at McDonald's? You can still have a burger if you don't eat the bun. You can also eat the hamburger fixings and even add cheese and avocado. You just can't have ketchup.

To determine if you're missing out, research is key. Consulting resources like a nutritionist can help you make sure you're getting all of the necessary vitamins and minerals while on the keto diet.

The Cons of Following a Keto Diet

Let's go back to the women who didn't stay on the diet in the case study I mentioned earlier. We don't know the reasons they quit, but it's easy to imagine some of the hardships of following a keto diet. What do you do if your lifestyle does not fit into the keto diet? What if you work long hours and rarely have time to shop for food or to prepare it? Eating out on keto is possible, but you have to be really clever and form habits like ordering hamburgers without buns and ordering subway sandwiches as salads. But what if all your boss will spring for on those late nights at the office is pizza? How do you stay on keto then? Well, I guess you'd have to scrape everything off the crust and be happy to eat a globby mess?

If you can't keep yourself in ketosis, the whole diet thing just fails. If you aren't getting your body to burn fat, you aren't going to be losing a lot of weight. With any diet, it is about what feels right for you. Moreover, finding a lifestyle change that you can follow is also important. If the keto diet sounds right for you, by all means, follow it. But if it doesn't sound right, know that there are other options out there. Skip ahead to see the other diet options available to find one that will fit your lifestyle.

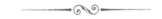

CHAPTER SUMMARY

● The keto diet's macronutrient pyramid states that you can eat 75% fat, 20% protein, and 5% carbs.

● Ketosis is the metabolic state of burning stored fat instead of glucose.

● The keto diet is more about what you can eat as opposed to what you can't.

In the next chapter, you will learn about the right mindset for dieting.

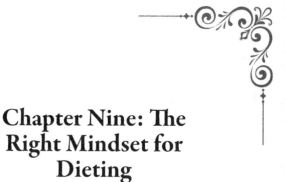

Chapter Nine: The Right Mindset for Dieting

It is clearly necessary to control your blood sugar and the amount of insulin that your body produces to reverse insulin sensitivity. Once the insulin sensitivity is under control, you have a huge chance to reverse the symptoms of PCOS. Without an overdose of insulin in your body, your ovaries will not have any reason to make more testosterone, and from there, you have the means to change your life. But how do you get into a mindset that will bring about positive change in your eating habits? I offer you 35 life hacks to get into the right mindset for dieting.

35 Mind Hacks for the Positive Attitude of Change

1. **Dig deep**. Decide that you want to do something about your PCOS. Do you want to reverse the damaging effects of having too many androgens in your system? Do you want to increase your chances of fertility? Find that reason that gives you the energy to set a goal. Be quantitative with your goal. Don't just say I want to lose weight. Be definite and decide what you want to happen and how long it will take you to get that done.

2. **Gather data**. Analyze the pros and cons of several diet plans. Write down the outcome of any diets that you have tried in the past. What was your success rate? What would you do differently? Ask yourself any questions that will help you to decide what is best for you.

3. **Make a decision** based on the data you have collected. Choose the diet/meal plan that is best for you.

4. **Find a mentor**, a coach or a support group that will be a positive influence in your life. For example, I find doing exercise exceedingly difficult. So, I chose a coach who loves to exercise, so I could learn from her what it takes to be an active person. Find support among your friends. You'd be surprised at how many people are struggling to lose weight. Find the person who has lost the most weight and find out what they did to succeed. Then, adopt some of the same habits.

5. **Train your brain**. Sometimes you must be mindful and concentrate to make every experience count. Get rid of any negative thoughts that you have about dieting and exercise. Rethink the process of losing weight. See the gains as an opportunity to learn how to diet better. When you lose weight, focus on the actions that brought you success.

6. **Find techniques that work for you.** Is it helpful for you to track all the food you eat? Do you like to try new recipes on a weekly or daily basis? Does developing a routine help you to stick to your diet? You need to explore the techniques that help you to stay on your healthy eating/diet plan and stick with the ones that work for you.

7. **Be your own best friend.** Don't be afraid to encourage yourself to do well. The more positive you are with yourself, the

more successful you will be. Believe that you can make the right choices for your healthy eating plan.

8. **Measure your success without the scale**. What's in a number? There are other ways to measure your success. For instance, keep track of how you feel physically and emotionally. Don't be afraid to make other assessments besides the scale.

9. **Take your time.** Remember that you are on your own time. Do not rush or compare yourself to someone else. Have your own timeline for getting better.

10. **Identify your trouble areas.** What is the hardest thing for you to do? Is it tracking your food or following your meal plan? Or is it exercise that's more difficult? When you isolate what is the trickiest thing for you to do, you can make a goal or strategy to make things easier on yourself.

11. **Imagine your success.** Be extremely specific in imagining your success. Think of the things you want to improve. See yourself improving, and you will see success. Think of how you will feel and the things you need to do to get there. Let loose with your imagination.

12. **Control is yours.** There is no one but you to make decisions and implement things. You have total control over the things you choose to do. No one else can push you into anything.

13. **Work with your emotions.** Are there any issues that you deal with by eating? Concentrate on that issue and develop a strategy for dealing with that emotion in a different way. If you eat when you are sad, try taking a walk or talking to your support person. Work with your feelings to resolve emotional eating.

14. **Organize your life**. Things are simply better when you organize whether you are mapping out your schedule, your physical stuff, or even the way you deal with your new health plan/diet. Get rid of emotional clutter, and you will find that things will get easier for you.

15. **Clean out your kitchen**. Do you still have food in your refrigerator and pantry that can sabotage your new healthy eating plan? Do you have food in any of your other rooms? Give away or throw away the items that are going to compromise your new plan.

16. **Prepare your food ahead of time.** You will be able to deal with your menu plan a lot better if you prepare things ahead of time. Chop vegetables and fruit and pre-cook to save yourself time later. It's easier to have a good attitude when you have the little things taken care of.

17. **Dress for the part.** Remember when you played dress-up as a kid and pretended to be a princess or a superhero? "Faking it until you make it" can go a long way when you're changing your lifestyle. The more you think "new" thoughts and plan new strategies, the closer you will be to your goal. It's all about becoming.

18. **Write a list.** You can't change things if you don't know what needs to change. Write a list and work on carrying out everything on that list. Take it one step at a time, and break down what you want to do into simple chunks of action.

19. **Find a time to be quiet.** With all the noise of daily life, it is impossible to really "hear" what's going on inside. Take a moment to be still, and clear your mind. You will find this makes you stronger and more focused.

20. **Get rid of old habits.** Write a list of the unhealthy habits that you want to get rid of and be mindful of the areas of your life where these unhealthy habits cause you trouble. One by one, replace these unhealthy habits with better habits to help you reach your goals.

21. **Daily affirmations.** Pick a good affirmation and repeat it to yourself daily. For example, you could say to yourself, "I will be successful in every way." You can make your own affirmation or look online for something that really resonates with you.

22. **Focus on the big picture.** When you have a difficult day or you find some of your routines challenging, think of the positive outcomes that your new routines will bring to you. Don't forget that your new health plan/diet is going to lift you out of the doldrums and into a better life. Do whatever it takes to stay focused on the big picture.

23. **Pick one small task to focus on.** Sometimes, trying a bunch of new things at one time can be daunting. Instead of doing a whole bunch of new things, pick one small thing and get busy with it. It could be taking a walk or drinking more water. Pick one and concentrate on doing it well.

24. **Journal your thoughts and ideas.** A journal can help clear your mind of its clutter and it can be a good outlet for your emotions. Right down the things that you want to improve and your feelings about the changes that are going on in your life. Try out innovative ideas in your journal and channel your fear onto paper so that you can bring them out into the light of your consciousness.

25. **Celebrate your changes and challenges.** Each Day that you overcome a challenge or make a positive change, you

must celebrate. Pat yourself on the back or reward yourself by doing something healthy and fun. Changing your lifestyle to be healthy and lose weight is a big accomplishment. Take the time to celebrate your challenging work.

26. **Schedule fun into your day.** Pick something fun to do every day. Whether it is finding a new joke to tell your family and share a laugh, or taking the time to skip like you are a child again. The more fun you incorporate into your life, the happier you will be.

27. **Ask the tough questions.** When you fight with yourself to do something, ask the tough questions of yourself to get to the core of what is making you fight against trying new and healthy behaviors.

28. **Get a good night's sleep.** Stick to a bedtime hygiene plan so that you can fall asleep at times that will allow you to get eight good hours of sleep. Don't skip your nighttime routine to watch a movie or do something that will get you into bed late.

29. **Take the long way.** Don't be afraid to take the long route to get to where you are going. Park your car far enough away so that you can take more steps. Don't be afraid to start moving more and walking more when you do things. Practical movement is just as good as purposeful movement. In other words, the walk through the parking lot is just as helpful as the mile you walk on a treadmill.

30. **Make the better choice.** When choosing your meal or organizing your time, make the better choice instead of the easier one. It is just as easy to reach for an apple as it is a cookie. It is just as easy to do five minutes of stretching to relax than sitting for ten minutes doing nothing.

31. **Identify your triggers.** What are the things that trigger you into making some not so good choices? If you isolate your triggers, you can begin to dismantle them and render them unsuccessful in getting you off track.

32. **Drink your water.** Make this your next good habit to learn. When you are losing weight, water is so important for you. Start out slow with the water consumption and then work yourself up to a healthy amount of daily water drinking.

33. **Keep a food diary.** If you have a smartphone or camera, snap a picture of what you are eating. Do this for a week and you will have concrete evidence of making good choices for yourself. Also, you will be able to refer to the pictures when you want to plan meals for the future.

34. **Mindful eating.** Eating in a calm, peaceful environment is much more beneficial to your mood than eating in front of the computer or television. Be mindful of the meal that you are eating.

35. **Be grateful.** Giving gratitude is the most positive thing you can do for yourself in your day. When we are grateful, we stress the importance of what we are doing and are thankful for our successes.

This is an extensive list of things to do. Don't try to do them all in one day. The most important thing is to change your mindset and think positive. Go through this list and choose the things you would like to do on a daily basis. Try each new thing with patience and understanding. Do not force yourself to do things that are too difficult to do. Slowly come to an understanding with yourself that change can be difficult but is possible.

By changing the way you think, you can make great strides in your personal life to be healthier and to lose the weight that needs to come off. Changing your diet can result in tremendous changes in your health. Do not be afraid to embrace these new healthy habits. They might be scary at first, but when you give them a chance, they will get easier and easier to do each day.

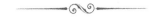

CHAPTER SUMMARY

• Having the right mindset for dieting is very important to the success of your diet.

• Focusing on the positive aspects of your healthy eating plan is essential to restoring your health.

• Changing your diet in order to be healthy can have a tremendous impact on your PCOS.

In the next chapter, you will learn about the PCOS diet.

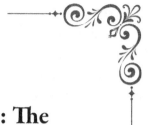

Chapter Ten: The PCOS Diet

U p to this point in the book, we have discussed the importance of healthy diets, including the anti-inflammatory diet and the keto diet. We have also learned about the glycemic index. All these diets can help with the symptoms of PCOS. The theory is that anything that can help with insulin resistance and inflammation is going to help or even reverse PCOS. The following are recommendations for the PCOS Diet, a way of eating specifically designed for women with PCOS.

Drink More Water

There are several different recommendations for the amount of water you should drink. Some say eight 8 ounce glasses of water is vital. Others say to drink 1 ½ ounces of water per pound.

Water helps your body function. Specifically, water helps your hormonal systems to work at peak performance and helps your glands secrete the right number of hormones. Also, water does many things, but at its most important, it helps the liver get rid of toxins.

Limit your tea, coffee, and alcohol intake. These drinks elevate your blood-sugar levels, and this in turn raises your insulin levels.

Increase the Amount of Fruit and Vegetables That You Eat Daily

Fruits and vegetables are sources of antioxidants, vitamins, minerals, and phytochemicals. Vegetables high in phytochemicals have compounds that help lower excessive androgen levels that are found in women who have PCOS.

The best thing to do is to create a "rainbow" of fruits and vegetables on your plate so that you will get the vast and varied vitamins, minerals, and phytochemicals that are present in fruits and vegetables.

Another reason to eat fruits and vegetables is that they contain fiber and fiber helps to lower your elevated blood sugar levels. In turn, this lowers your insulin levels so your ovaries won't be inclined to produce more androgens.

Eat Complex Carbohydrates

Again, women who have PCOS may suffer from insulin resistance, so giving your body a carbohydrate that is low on the glycemic index is a good thing because it will help with your blood sugar level.

50% of your diet can come from carbohydrates so that you can provide your body with food that converts to energy. Choosing carbs that are complex is the best thing for a woman with PCOS and insulin resistance.

Chapter Five talks more about the glycemic index and glycemic loads.

Remember that sugar is a carbohydrate that gets absorbed quickly and one that can play havoc with your blood sugar. It isn't enough to just stay away from items like cupcakes and cookies, you also must pay attention to hidden sugars like those in commercial pasta sauces, breakfast cereals, and fruit drinks.

Also, it isn't enough to just stay away from sugar, but you also must be careful of honey, molasses, dextrose, glucose, fructose, maltose, corn syrup, and industrial sugars that are added to processed foods.

Fiber is Your Friend

For a woman with PCOS and insulin resistance, fiber helps to keep your blood sugar from getting too high. For example, sweetened applesauce will immediately get digested and consequently, your blood sugar will soar. However, if you eat an apple, the fiber in that apple will slow down digestion and your blood sugar will stay low.

Another reason for eating foods high in fiber is it helps your body get rid of toxins and built-up hormones as it pushes through your system.

A good amount of fiber is 30-50 grams. Also, make sure to drink your water to help the fiber pass through your system.

How Much Protein Should You Eat in a Day?

There is a formula for deciding how much protein you need:

The suggestion is 0.8 grams of protein per kilogram of body weight or 0.36 per pound (Groves, 2018).

If you are sedentary, you might need 46 grams per day. If you are active, you might need more. In the end, you can decide how much protein that you need.

Eat the best protein that you can find. You might not want to eat steak, but how about a nice boiled egg or even a good piece of cheese? There is no shame in eating foods like peanut butter, but make sure the brand you pick doesn't have some of that hidden sugar we've been talking about.

Protein is important because it keeps your blood sugar balanced and helps to supply your body with amino acids. Amino acids are important because they build and repair cells and create hormones.

Our bodies can store amino acids, so you have to supply your body with the proteins it needs to create them.

For a woman with PCOS, protein is especially important because it stimulates the production of glucagon. Glucagon is important because it helps your body use stored fat as a fuel source. When your body can use a glucagon as an energy source, it does not need to use so much glucose. This means that your body does not need to put so much insulin into your system. And you guessed it, this process helps with insulin sensitivity.

Protein also builds up your muscles and this can help you burn more calories. Consequently, it will reverse the effect that PCOS has on making weight loss difficult.

While you are filling half of your plate with the rainbow of fruits and vegetables, try to get two portions of carbs for every one portion of protein.

Don't Forget About Fatty Acids (EFAs)

PCOS is associated with the metabolism of fatty acids. You need essential fats to "regulate hormone function and strengthen cell walls" (Morris, 2011). When you have enough fat in your diet, this increases your chances of a regular menstrual cycle.

20-25% of your calories from fat should go towards your total calories in a 2,000 calorie a day diet. This comes to about 44-77 grams.

High quality fats help slow down the entry of carbohydrates and this helps your insulin sensitivity by helping to stabilize your blood sugar.

When you have stable blood sugar, your mental health improves, and you have a better ability to focus. PCOS symptoms are also not so detrimental.

EFAs are essential fatty acids that you find in omega-3 or omega-6 rich foods. You need these ESAs to help produce hormones like ovarian and stress hormones. If you don't get enough ESAs, this can affect your ability to ovulate.

Eat More Phytonutrients

Phytonutrients or phytochemicals are found naturally in plants. These are the chemicals that give plants color and flavor.

Phytonutrients are important to fight against the symptoms of PCOS. They are as significant as vitamins and minerals in keeping you healthy. They do things like preventing heart disease, memory loss, and they reduce the risk of diabetes.

Phytonutrients are also known to keep your reproductive health in decent shape.

It isn't necessary to go on a big hunt to find foods with phytonutrients because every fruit and vegetable has phytonutrients. It isn't enough to just eat fruits and vegetables – eating a variety is also important. A good rule of thumb is to create a rainbow of color with fruit. Why just eat apples and oranges when you can also eat peaches, melons, and all sorts of berries? Vegetables such as the different colored bell peppers, carrots, and cabbage can put more phytonutrients in your body.

There are distinct groups of phytochemicals, such as flavonoids, that help to prevent heart disease and strokes. Phytoestrogens help lower the risk of breast cancer and carotenoids protect against heart disease, cancer, and Alzheimer's disease (Briden, 2018).

Keep Your Cholesterol Low

Cholesterol isn't as bad as it has been made out to be over the years. It helps with the creation of sex hormones like estrogen and progesterone and other bodily processes, but it is true that you can have too much of it, and that's not good.

Also of concern is that the contraceptive pill you may have been prescribed for PCOS can lower your HDL and increase you LDL levels.

So, what does this mean?

There is good cholesterol HDL (high-density lipoprotein) and bad cholesterol LDL (low density lipoprotein). HDL transports excess amounts of LDL out of your system.

Back to the situation with your birth control pills. The fact that it lowers HDL means that there probably won't be enough of it to transport all the LDL in your system, so that is why LDL levels increase when you are on the pill.

Another cholesterol fact is that women with PCOS have a 7x higher risk of having a heart attack than women who do not have PCOS (Briden, 2018).

So, how can you help your body get rid of LDL?

Well, you can exercise, but you can also step up your consumption of garlic and oily fish like herring, mackerel, sardines, tuna and salmon because these foods contain omega-3 and this helps the body get rid of LDL. Fruits and vegetables help lower cholesterol. Olive oil, kidney beans, chickpeas, soy-based foods also lower your levels of LDL (Briden, 2018).

Fiber also aids your body in the excretion of LDL. Substantial amounts of fat are kept from being absorbed if you have fiber in your system.

Red wine can also help lessen your LDL levels because it has an antioxidant that is known to decrease cholesterol.

Reduce Your Salt Intake

Instead of adding salt to your diet, try some tasty alternatives via your spice rack.

Women with PCOS are 4x are more susceptible to high blood pressure. Consuming a lot of salt can retain fluids, and this raises your blood pressure.

Have you ever wondered what exactly blood pressure is and why it's always distinguished by two numbers?

First of all, the force of the blood against the inner walls of your blood vessels is what health professionals measure. This is called your blood pressure. The systolic and diastolic value is what gives you those two numbers.

Systolic value stands for "the force that the heart pumps blood through your body." The diastolic value is the "pressure of the blood vessels when they are relaxed (McCulloch, 2016).

The upper number is the systolic number and the lower number is the diastolic number.

A normal blood pressure reading for a woman is 120/80. It's the bottom number that is important to watch because anything over 90 is considered to be high, and therefore hypertensive.

If your blood pressure is high, you are at risk for heart disease, stroke, and kidney problems. You can take prescribed medication to lower your blood pressure but your lifestyle and what you eat can also lower the diastolic value of your blood pressure.

If you have a healthy diet, you will lower your risk of high blood pressure. But the thing to really watch out for is your consumption of salt. A healthy limit for salt is 5 grams per day. You can cut down on the salt you shake onto your meals, and even better, you can limit the amount of salt you use when you cook.

The real problem comes with the foods that are high in salt like in cured, smoked, or canned meats. Any food that is processed or salty should be viewed with caution. Foods that are high in salt can cause you to exceed your personal salt limit.

Use other ways to put flavor in your food instead of salt. Herbs like basil, dill and fennel can enhance a meal. Garlic is another flavor enhancer to use when you are cooking. Even wine can add flavor to your food.

Changing Your Lifestyle

There is no shame in needing a specific food plan that will help lower your insulin production. Following the guidelines in this chapter will lead you towards a healthy lifestyle. The important thing to remember is changing your lifestyle is a necessary step in reversing your PCOS.

When adopting a new diet, keep your symptoms in mind. Make changes that will alleviate your symptoms while also addressing the root causes of this syndrome: insulin resistance and inflammation. A diet consisting of complex carbs, vegetables, fruits, healthy fats, and proteins has been shown to be effective for many women with PCOS. It can be for you too.

If you already follow a healthy diet, that's wonderful. Continue on it, and let your doctor or nurse practitioner know that you are following healthy guidelines for your nutrition.

As always, seek medical attention for evaluation of your diet and to know if you do have insulin resistance or sensitivity. Your doctor or nurse practitioner can recommend the appropriate test that will show exactly how resistant you are to insulin.

Above all, don't lose faith that you can take control of your life and make a difference in your health.

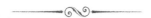

CHAPTER SUMMARY

- There is no specific PCOS diet.

- Following certain nutritional guidelines can influence your meal plan.

- A PCOS diet is one that directly addresses the nutritional needs of reversing the symptoms of PCOS.

If you are enjoying this book, please consider leaving it a review!

In the next chapter, you will learn about PCOS and the vegan diet.

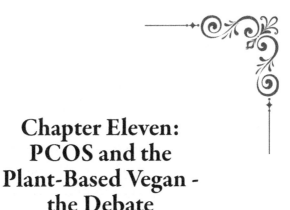

Chapter Eleven:
PCOS and the
Plant-Based Vegan -
the Debate

O f all the diet plans circulating in popular literature, the vegan diet is touted as being the healthiest food plan available to women with PCOS. There are benefits to eating a plant-based diet but when such diets are scrutinized, there are deficits that can't be ignored.

Typically, a plant-based diet focuses on not eating any processed foods or animal products. It is a diet rich in fresh vegetables, fruits, legumes, beans, nuts, seeds, and whole grains. On the surface, it seems that a vegan diet would be plant-based, but there are differences.

For example, grocery shelves are filled with vegan packaged snacks and vegan "meats" that are made with beans, legumes, and whole wheat. There are noodles and pastas that do not have any ingredients that would make a vegan cringe. Yet, these foods are not necessarily healthy. In fact, we can make an argument that these vegan convenience foods are one step away from being processed foods.

Not all vegans buy into the special vegan foods that are sold at grocery stores. There are many that stay close to a plant-based diet and all the wholesome foods that go with it. They not only eat whole foods, but they also include alternative supplements that add the vitamins and minerals that they miss out on by not eating any animal products.

For the sake of argument, I will be comparing a plant-based vegan diet to a basic PCOS diet. Specifically, I will not be writing about the vegan diet that includes convenience foods. Also, I will be referring to an article by nutritionist Robyn Srigley called "3 Benefits of Plant-Based Eating for PCOS" as my source for this discussion about plant-based veganism.

The Goals of Any PCOS Diet

The goal of any woman with PCOS is to address insulin resistance and other issues like excess androgens. Can a plant-based vegan diet fit the profile of a diet that helps counter the symptoms of PCOS? Moreover, is a plant based vegan diet superior to any other diet that has been discussed in this book?

A Mineral and Vitamin Rich Diet

A diet of plant-based food brings with it many different vitamins and minerals. For example, if you eat dark leafy green vegetables, like kale and spinach, you will be consuming B vitamins, folate, vitamin C, magnesium, calcium, and manganese.

A health tip often given by nutritionists is to arrange a rainbow of colors on your plate when eating fruits and vegetables because this guarantees that you will be eating a variety of nutrient-dense foods.

Eating nutrient dense vegetables and fruits supplies a replenishment of nutritional deficiencies found in PCOS. These nutrients help reduce inflammation and help with insulin resistance.

A PCOS Detox

When you are eating a plant-based vegan diet, you are cleansing and detoxifying your body in a way that no other diet can claim. The anti-inflammatory phytonutrients in plant-based food, fiber, vitamins, and minerals, go a long way in detoxifying your body.

Fiber, especially, will lead the charge in pushing toxins from your liver out of your body. This is important because with PCOS, you have a lot of excess build-up of hormones. Anything that can help these hormones exit your body is an incredibly good thing.

When your body is flooded with nutrients, your detox organs (liver, lungs, kidneys, colon) can work more effectively to remove toxins from your system.

Fiber in the Plant-Based Diet

There are three ways that the fiber in a plant-based vegan diet addresses the fight to reverse the effects of PCOS. Fiber binds with excess estrogen, fiber is good for probiotics and fiber helps to regulate insulin and blood sugar.

When you have PCOS, you have an excess of estrogen in your system. It is ideal to have something that can help remove that excess estrogen before it does something damaging. Fiber is the key to removing excess estrogen because fiber binds with estrogen and escorts it out of the body through our digestive system. When estrogen is balanced, you have a higher likelihood of a normal menstrual cycle and some of your other PCOS symptoms like heavy facial and body hair begin to improve.

Another benefit to the high fiber content of a vegan plant-based diet is that fiber feeds the probiotics that are in our system. A probiotic that balances estrogen is estrobolome and fiber feeds it so that it can do its job.

Lastly, the top job for fiber is to help regulate insulin and blood sugar. When you balance a meal with fiber, protein, and fat, you put food into your system that isn't going to spike your blood sugar. Fiber in any carbohydrate makes it a complex carbohydrate and therefore it's slow to be absorbed into our systems.

Consequently, a fiber rich diet can help with insulin resistance and weight loss. Two of the most important processes that help to reverse the symptoms of PCOS.

The Downfalls of a Plant-Based Vegan Diet

The three benefits of a plant-based vegan diet are pretty valuable to PCOS, but the same things can be accomplished in a less radical way by following other diets, such as the keto diet or the anti-inflammatory diet. In fact, following the guidelines for a good PCOS diet also ensures that you get your fiber and nutrients-filled fruits and vegetables. So, it doesn't take the sacrifice of not having animal products in your diet to achieve positive results.

A big drawback to not having animal products in your diet is that you lose some of the nutrients like B12 and amino acids that can only be found in these types of food. Yes, you can take supplements, but they won't be able to add the high amounts of vitamins and amino acids that our bodies need.

A vegan diet is high in carbs by nature. When you remove animal products from your diet, there exists a vacuum that is filled with carbohydrates. In order for a vegan to get their portion of protein into their diet, they often rely on high protein plant-based foods that are also high in carbohydrates.

Following the strict guidelines of a plant-based vegan diet can be stressful, and at times inconvenient. When you go vegan, there are so many restrictions on your diet. Not being able to have cheese, milk, eggs or other foods that are readily available, often leads a person to buy vegan convenience foods that have none of the benefits that lead a person to follow a plant-based vegan diet in the first place.

A Few Positives About Plant-based Vegan Diets

There is a concern that eating animal products like beef, pork, poultry, butter and cheese raises your consumption of the highly reactive molecules called AGEs (advanced glycation end products). When these foods are cooked at a high temperature, there are even more AGEs released.

AGEs are not good for women with PCOS because these highly reactive molecules can induce inflammation, cellular damage, and insulin resistance. This isn't good when you are trying to choose foods and follow a meal plan that is going to help relieve symptoms of your PCOS.

Diets, such as the keto diet, that encourage the consumption of high fat and protein levels, may increase the amount of AGEs that you get in your diet.

Foods that are low in AGEs are whole grains, legumes, vegetables, and fruits. So, you can make an argument that when you follow a plant-based vegan diet, you will not be adding AGEs to your diet.

Soy and PCOS

In a 2018 randomized trial, 60 women with PCOS were divided into two groups where one group had more soy protein than the other. The group that had soy proteins lost more weight and cut down on insulin resistance (Karamali, 2018).

Vegans who follow a plant-based diet are more prone to getting their protein from products that contain soy. Soy products like tofu, tempeh and soy milk are considered to be complete proteins, so these are good choices for a vegan. Soy also helps vegans get more essential amino acids not in their diet.

One could conclude that since soy has a positive effect on women with PCOS, the plant-based vegan diet is more favorable.

A 2017 study published in *Diabetes and Metabolic Syndrome: Clinical Research & Reviews* reported that a diet that is low in saturated fatty acids and high in fiber is good for women with PCOS. Again, a vegan plant-based diet that is mostly whole grains, legumes, vegetables, and fruits is highly recommended. However, the key to this study is that the carbohydrates in this diet had to be low on the glycemic index, something that carbs on vegan plant-based diets often are not (McMaken, 2017).

Health Benefits of Plant Based Diets for PCOS

When a person is arguing that plant-based vegan diets are better for women with PCOS, they often will cite the health benefits that this diet promotes. Women with PCOS have a problem with insulin resistance, chronic inflammation, altered gut microbiomes. and elevated androgens (McMaken, 2017). The benefits of a plant-based vegan diet seems to correct or help these problems.

The positive attributes of a plant-based vegan diet are decreased insulin resistance, cholesterol levels, and inflammation. Vegans also enjoy a healthier gut microbiome and weight loss.

However, there is a clear downside to a plant-based vegan diet: you have to prop up this diet with alternative supplements to get vitamin B12, calcium, iron, omega 3s, and choline.

However, a plant-based vegan diet has the added benefit of being rich in nutrients like vitamin B6 and vitamin C, folate, potassium, magnesium, phosphorus, and beta-carotene.

The Staying Power of a Plant-Based Vegan Diet

The bottom line for any diet that is going to help with PCOS is the period of time that a woman spends on this diet. An initial period of four weeks or a month is the average for a woman staying on a diet, but is this long enough to have an impact on PCOS? A long-term diet plan is going to be more beneficial for improving your PCOS symptoms, but what is it going to take for you to stay on a diet? The plant-based vegan diet, theoretically, sounds great. You've got fiber and nutrient-dense foods to be excited about. Filling your plate with a rainbow of fruits and vegetables can not only be visually stimulating, but it can also stimulate your palate and make you feel mentally good about yourself for eating so healthy.

But what is going to happen when you start missing animal products? Will it happen? Can your craving for meat by satisfied by a plate full of vegetables? One can argue that you can buy an assortment of vegan products that simulate meat, but will these products be as nutritious as actual beef? And, most especially, do these products still adhere to the guidelines of a plant-based vegan diet?

A lot of times when a person chooses to be a vegan, they have non-food motives. They can choose to not eat animal products based on environmental reasons or their love for animals. Eating vegan can be about the ethics of not eating anything that has a face.

A person that is vegan often makes a moral statement with what she chooses to eat. Food choices become all about what the vegan believes in and what she supports. Perhaps it is all of this emotion that keeps a vegan on her plant-based diet.

What happens when you are following a plant-based vegan diet for health reasons only? Will you have the gumption to stick to it?

The number one issue is you must stick to a diet for a significant period of time to be able to reap the benefits. If you are following a diet that is hard to be compliant on, you may not get the health benefits that you need.

Life happens to the best of us and there will be days when you aren't prepared to eat on the run. You go off your plant-based vegan diet and eat something that is not on your diet. This begins to happen, once, twice, and maybe three times, and then where are you in your healthy eating recovery plan?

A plant-based vegan diet is high on some nutrition benefits but low on convenience and practicality. You can still reap the benefits of a plant-based vegan diet without having to make the sacrifices a vegan makes. Healthy eating so often includes healthy portions of nutrition-dense fruits and vegetables and complex carbohydrates. Proteins from animal products are eaten in healthy portions. In the end, a plant-based vegan diet asks for too many sacrifices that lead to an incompatibility with real life.

CHAPTER SUMMARY

● A plant-based vegan diet has many qualities that can benefit women with PCOS.

● It is hard to stay on a vegan diet because of all the things you can not eat.

● It is much easier to follow another type of diet and still get the same results as you would if you followed a vegan diet.

In the next chapter, you will learn about alternative supplements that can help with the symptoms of PCOS.

Chapter Twelve:
Additional
Supplements and
Medications

There are many people who will defend alternative medicine as being legitimate and really helping to alleviate the symptoms of an illness. Some of these same people will even goes as far as saying that alternative medicine can cure an illness when a prescribed medication can't.

In the case of PCOS, there are alternative medications that seem to be making a difference. What follows is a list of supplements or alternative medicines that have been shown to help the many different symptoms of PCOS.

Although it is tempting to go buy these supplements and administer them yourself, this list is in no way comprehensive enough to tell you how to take these supplements in a way that's safe and effective. It is recommended that you see a doctor who specializes in PCOS and is familiar with these supplements and how they work.

The following is a guide that you can use when you consult a health professional about PCOS and the alternative supplements and medications that treat it.

Magnesium

Magnesium, the chemical element that is represented as MG and has an atomic number of 12, has been at the forefront of supplements that are given to women with PCOS.

Magnesium seems to help with insulin resistance and thus, decreasing the chances of developing diabetes. As you know, insulin resistance is at the core of PCOS. So, being able to take something that can help with insulin resistance is a big deal.

Other symptoms that magnesium helps with include anxiety, blood pressure, PMS symptoms, and sleep.

The way magnesium helps with anxiety is by calming the nervous system and preventing excessive creation of cortisol, the stress hormone. The adrenal glands make cortisol and magnesium supports this production. When stress happens, magnesium runs low because it's helping the adrenal glands with its production of cortisol (Grassi, 2019).

There are different types of magnesium on the market: magnesium glycinate (magnesium malate product), magnesium citrate, magnesium gluconate, magnesium orotate, and magnesium aspartate. Be cautious of taking magnesium oxide because it is hard to absorb and often causes diarrhea. Also, magnesium citrate should only be taken when you are constipated as it may produce loose stools. The recommended dose for magnesium is 400-600 mg per day. It is also recommended that you take calcium in a ratio of 2:1 calcium to magnesium (Grassi, 2019).

Foods that are high in magnesium are:

- Seeds: pumpkin seeds, sunflower seeds, and sesame seeds

- Nuts: almonds and hazelnuts
- Legumes: peanuts, black beans, and soybeans
- Whey protein
- Grains: rice, oats, sorghum, barley, and teff
- Vegetables: spinach and potatoes
- Raw cacao

Vitamin D

If you have PCOS, it is important for your healthcare provider to check your levels of vitamin D. If you are deficient, there will be a need for you to take vitamin D as a supplement. In two different studies, vitamin D was shown to improve menstrual regularity and increase fertility.

Vitamin D is known for its role in hormonal balance and immunities. Healthcare professionals are careful about the amount of vitamin D that they recommend because the vitamin is known to cling to the walls of your arteries, causing them to harden. Doctors often prescribe vitamin K and vitamin A to help curb this risk.

The *Journal of Obstetrics & Gynecology* did a study with infertile PCOS women who took 1000 milligrams of calcium and 400 international (IU) per day of vitamin D. At the end of three months, the women reported improvements in their menstrual regularity. Vitamin D and calcium can help regulate your menstrual cycles and help you ovulate.

The *European Journal of Endocrinology* did a study with women who had PCOS and were infertile. The results of the study showed the women in the study had more mature follicles, making them more likely to get pregnant. The women who did not take vitamin D had less mature follicles and therefore, a lower chance of getting pregnant.

Other studies have reported that vitamin D not only improves fertility, but it also lowers testosterone levels and inflammation (Grassi, 2018).

Foods that are high in vitamin D are fortified dairy products (milk, yogurt, etc.), eggs, liver, swordfish, salmon, tuna, and cod liver oil.

Zinc

Zinc is a chemical element that has been found to help improve fertility, counter the effects of excess testosterone, and reduce inflammation in when taken with magnesium.

A study by Biological Trace Elements Research gave 50 mg of zinc daily to one group of women and a placebo to another. All of the women had PCOS. After eight weeks, 41.7% of the women had significantly less hair loss compared to the women who took the placebo. Also, these women saw a reduction in hair growth related to hirsutism.

Zinc is known to be part of hair follicles and can keep hair from falling out while it also stimulating hair to grow. Therefore, researchers are interested in how it works with women who have PCOS and have issues with hair loss and excessive hair growth.

The *Journal of Obstetrics and Gynecology Research* tested women with PMS by giving them 50 mg of Zinc during the last two weeks of their menstrual cycle. The women who did not take the placebo had a significant rise in their quality of life and experienced an improvement in their symptoms of PMS.

Some medical theorists believe that zinc binds to insulin and helps insulin to get glucose into cells. PCOS women who are insulin resistant have low levels of zinc, while PCOS women who do not have trouble with insulin have higher levels of zinc (Grassi, 2017).

It's also important to note that birth control pills are known to deplete zinc levels (Grassi, 2017). That said, zinc has been shown to improve fertility and reduce the effects of high testosterone levels in women with PCOS.

Foods that are high in Zinc are:

- Shellfish, particularly oysters
- Meat: beef, bison, lamb, and turkey
- Legumes: black beans, azuki beans
- Seeds: pumpkin and sunflower

Chromium

Chromium is a chemical element that helps metabolize sugar. This in turn helps stabilize insulin resistance. Chromium can also improve you body mass index (Grassi, 2017).

B12

Vitamin B12 is known for its role in red blood cell formation, DNA synthesis, and nerve function. Moreover, B12 may improve fertility and fatigue in women with PCOS (Groves, 2018).

Foods high in vitamin B12 are:

- Shellfish: mussels, oysters and crabs
- Fish: herring and salmon
- Meat: liver, beef and pork
- Eggs
- Dairy products: milk and yogurt

Folate or B9

Folate is different from folic acid. Folate is the vitamin B9 and folic acid is the synthetic form of B9. Folate is known to improve blood sugar and lipid levels. It also lowers inflammatory markers in women with PCOS (Groves, 2018). Folate and vitamin B 12 improve insulin resistance in patients with metabolic syndromes such as PCOS (Groves, 2018).

Foods high in folate are:

- Legumes: azuki beans, black beans, and soybeans

- Vegetables: asparagus, beets, spinach, broccoli, peas, cabbage, and collard greens.

The "B" Vitamins

One of the most important sets of vitamins to PCOS are the B vitamins: B2, B3, and B6. These vitamins aid in the correction of PCOS symptoms. They help the liver change old hormones into harmless substances that can be excreted from the body.

Some women with PCOS have problems with gaining too much weight. This occurs because they are insulin resistant. Vitamins B2, B3, B5 and B6 help the body control weight gain.

B2 helps by processing fat, sugar, and protein into energy.

B3 helps the body cope with rising levels of blood sugar by being a part of the glucose tolerance factor. In particular, B3 helps to keep glucose levels in balance.

B5 controls fat metabolism, which in turn helps the body lose weight.

B6 keeps hormones balanced.

B6, B2, and B3 are essential to normal thyroid hormone manufacturing. If these three hormones are out of balance, thyroid function is off, and this affects the metabolism – and therefore PCOS.

B8, inositol, like B3 also aids with fighting insulin resistance and supports fertility.

Vitamins and minerals are not the only alternatives to help reverse the symptoms of PCOS. There are lots of herbs and oils that can help.

When it comes to insulin resistance, there are several alternative choices that can help. Cinnamon, turmeric (curcumin) holy basil, licorice root and berberine, an herb used in Chinese medicine, all assist in preventing insulin resistance from happening.

When you are having trouble with your menstrual cycles and ovulation, there are a few herbal supplements you can turn to. Evening primrose can help with menstruation, while tribulus terrestris can also help with menstruation. It also stimulates ovulation and helps lessen the number of ovarian cysts found in women with PCOS. Chasteberry has been used for centuries to improve symptoms of PMS (Groves, 2018). Cod liver oil also helps with menstruation and with getting rid of fat around your waist.

Inflammation is sometimes a problem that is associated with PCOS, but turmeric and licorice root can help.

And, although not an herbal supplement, probiotics can reduce inflammation and even regulate the sex hormones.

There are two traditional herbs that can be used to help out with the symptoms of PCOS. Ashwagandha, also called the "Indian ginseng" balances out cortisol levels, improving stress and symptoms of PCOS such as the release of excess androgens (Groves, 2018). The Macca root is a traditional herb that improves fertility and libido. It also helps with depression.

Remember to use caution when you are taking herbal supplements because they have not been approved by the FDA. Always work with a health professional who is knowledgeable about alternative medicine.

Even though this chapter has been about alternative medicines, the reality is that it might be easier to take prescribed medicine because, let's face it, it is harder to find a doctor who is willing to supervise the use of alternative supplements. So, I am going to provide you with a list of medications that are used in the treatment of PCOS. It is good to know what these medications are used for. I am not going to use the trade names for these medications, but I will explain what the group of these drugs do to help with the management of PCOS.

The first group of medications treat the symptoms that are a byproduct of PCOS:

- Statins – reduces cholesterol synthesis so that the liver can remove circulating LDL cholesterol.

- Anti-hypertensives – drugs that treat hypertension (high blood pressure).

- Anti-depressants – drugs that help to increase the level of biogenic amines like norepinephrine, serotonin, and dopamine.

- Benzodiazepines – drugs that treat anxiety.

This second group of medications help to correct the symptoms of PCOS:

- Aromatase inhibitor – used in the treatment of infertility. This medication reduces the total amount of estrogen produced by the body.

- 5-alpha-reductase inhibitor – treats hirsutism by inhibiting the conversion of testosterone to DHT.

- Anti-androgenics – lowers excess androgens so that there is a decrease in hair loss (alopecia), acne, and abnormal hair growth on the face and body (hirsutism).

- Insulin sensitizing agent – management of irregular menstrual cycles, infertility, insulin resistance and hirsutism.

- Ovulation induction agent – works on the pituitary gland to release hormones that will stimulate ovulation.

- Oral contraceptives – management of menstrual irregularities and helps with excess facial and body hair (hirsutism).

Prescribed medications may be a godsend in the treatment of PCOS, but they also have some drawbacks. Here is a list (McCulloch, 2016) of some deficiencies that occur when taking these medications:

Folate depletion can happen when you take anti-depressants, Metformin, birth control pills, and Spironolactone.

The depletion of B12, B1 and vitamin A can occur when you take birth control pills and Metformin.

When you take birth control pills, you can have a depletion of magnesium and zinc. For more information on birth control, hormones, and other elements outside of diet that affect PCOS symptoms in a variety of ways, refer to the companion piece for this book, "PCOS, The New Science of Completely Reversing Symptoms," by myself, Jane Kennedy.

This book is not to be a substitute for medical advice. Those not seeing improvement can look to medications. Always consult your doctor for medical advice.

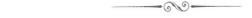

CHAPTER SUMMARY

- There are many natural supplements that help ease the symptoms of PCOS.

- There are medications that are used to curb the symptoms of PCOS.

- It is important to find a health professional that is an expert at knowing all about alternative supplements and the medicines that are given to treat PCOS.

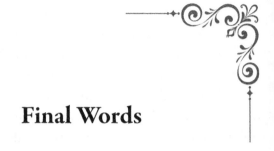

Final Words

I t seems like an impossible task, to reverse a metabolic syndrome that does not have an official cure. Yet, it can be done. Many women have done this by changing their lifestyle to include healthy eating. The nutrients contained in food have a way of healing us like no other substance can. The anti-inflammation diet, the keto diet, and the PCOS diet tips all have a place at the table when it comes to improving the health of women with PCOS. All these diets have healthy eating in common, even though they go about carrying out the same thing in different ways. The chapters in this book about these diets provides a good place to start. Overall, a healthy diet can really have a positive impact on your PCOS symptoms.

Learning lifestyle changes can also improve your symptoms. In this book, we discussed the glycemic index, diet breaks, the right mindset for dieting, and the role of exercise in the life of a woman with PCOS. Knowing the basics about the glycemic index is especially important to quashing insulin resistance. Eating foods with a low glycemic index helps to regulate the amount of insulin that is released into the bloodstream. Another important technique to learn is the taking of diet breaks to help with staying on a diet or food plan in the long term. Having the right mindset for dieting can be the difference between succeeding and failing. It is important to have a positive attitude to carry out something as tough as changing the way you eat. A good thought and the right goals can make all the difference. Finally, the role that exercise plays is especially important to a body that is dealing with PCOS. Developing habits that will help you lose weight is a major plus in trying to recover from the symptoms of PCOS.

There are distinct types of PCOS that show up in women. Not all women have the same symptoms, and this is important for treating PCOS. Not all women will have difficulty ovulating or a thick growth of hair. Yet, one trait that most women with PCOS share is insulin resistance. The inability of the cells to respond to insulin is a big problem that leads to some grave consequences. One of those consequences is excess androgens that cause a heavy growth of hair on the face and body, severe acne, and male pattern baldness.

Alternative remedies and supplements were explored in the last chapter to draw attention to the vitamins and minerals that can also be found in what you eat. When your diet does not give you what you need, it is good to have a back up plan. Supplements can provide this additional support. You should know about the different medications that are given to women with PCOS. It is important to consult with your doctor to know which medicines and supplements are better suited to the type of PCOS that you have.

In this book, I have tried to bring to you the information that I gathered from the latest scientific sources and research. Also, different testimonials from women with PCOS guided the writing of this book. PCOS is the most common metabolic syndrome in women. PCOS is also the leading cause of infertility in women. Not being able to ovulate is exceedingly difficult for many women. It is a hard symptom to deal with when you want to become a mother. Furthermore, symptoms like excess facial hair, severe weight gain, and male pattern baldness makes it hard to get through a regular day. Yet there is something you can do about your symptoms and that is to take charge of your diet and eat healthy.

If you take away just one thing from this book, I hope it is the feeling of empowerment. It isn't going to be easy to take charge of a syndrome like PCOS, but it can be done. The more you learn about PCOS, the more weapons you have to fight it. Weapons is an aggressive word, but perhaps, it is more important to get strong and fight PCOS and come out the other side feeling better and in charge of your life.

While doing my research, I was struck by the bravery of the women who have battled against the symptoms of PCOS. I found a Pinterest page filled with encouraging memes to fight against PCOS, and I even found out that PCOS has its own ribbon like breast cancer. The color of this ribbon is an incredibly beautiful shade of blue.

In the course of writing this book, I discovered by accident that I have a friend who has PCOS. I was at a school reunion, and I complimented her hair. You see, in all the pictures that I see of her on Facebook, she always has the most beautiful hair. She gave me a sad smile and admitted to me that she has alopecia and has actually lost the hair on her head. We then began to talk about PCOS, and she told me about the lifestyle changes that she had made over the course of a year. Finally, after struggling to find the right diet, she was beginning to see signs of improvement. She illustrated for me that even though PCOS is a widespread illness, the battle to reverse the symptoms of PCOS is a very personal thing and looks different for each woman. The diet that you choose must mean something to you. The choice to exercise comes down to a daily commitment to help your body burn calories more efficiently. My friend told me about her struggles, and she shared with me that it had been hard for her to find crucial information about PCOS. With this book, I hope that the women out there who need this information will find what they're looking for.

I would like to end this book with a quote from a meme that was very inspirational to me:

"When you are tempted to give up, your breakthrough is probably just around the corner."

- Joyce Meyer, PCOSLIVING.COM

I hope you enjoyed the content in this book and, most importantly, learned something that you can apply in your effort to live a better life with PCOS. If you are also interested in learning a collection of additional methods people are using to combat PCOS outside of dieting, please check out the companion book, PCOS – The New Science of Completely Reversing Symptoms, also written by me.

If you enjoyed this book, **please consider leaving a review!** This is a huge help for me and helps me to put out more content like this. Thanks for reading and good luck on your journey ahead!

References

Beat PCOS with Kym Campbell. (2019, September 27). Retrieved from https://beatpcos.com/

Briden, L. (2018). *Period repair manual: every woman's guide to better periods.* Sydney, N.S.W.: Macmillan.

Can you sing while you work out? (2019, August 6). Retrieved from https://www.mayoclinic.org/healthy-lifestyle/fitness/in-depth/exercise-intensity/art-20046887

Coyle, D. (2017, November 7). A Beginner's Guide to the Low-Glycemic Diet. Retrieved September 3, 2019, from https://www.healthline.com/nutrition/low-glycemic-diet.

Jean Hailes Foundation. (2011). *Evidence-based guideline for the assessment and management of polycystic ovary syndrome.* Clayton South, Victoria.

Futterweit, W., & Ryan, G. (2006). *A patients guide to Pcos: understanding and reversing polycystic ovarian syndrome.*

Galan, N. (2019, May 26). The Role Diet and Nutrition Play in PCOS Health. Retrieved from https://www.verywellhealth.com/vitamins-and-minerals-the-role-they-play-pcos-health-2616482

Glucophage (Metformin) and Diabetes. (0AD). Retrieved from https://www.diabetes.co.uk/diabetes-medication/glucophage.html

Grassi, A. (2018, February 28). 3 Reasons to Take Vitamin D If You Have PCOS. Retrieved from https://www.verywellhealth.com/vitamin-d-more-than-just-a-vitamin-2616313

Grassi, A. (2019, June 24). What Women With PCOS Should Know About Magnesium. Retrieved from https://www.verywellhealth.com/pcos-and-magnesium-4145000

Groves, M. (0AD). Post. Retrieved May 6, 2018, from https://www.avocadogrovenutrition.com/post/5-nutrients-for-women-with-pcos.

Gurevich, R. (2019, September 7). Androgens & PCOS: Excess Levels & What It Means. Retrieved from https://www.verywellhealth.com/androgens-and-pcos-excess-levels-what-it-means-4156771

Harris, C., & Francis-Cheung, T. (2016). *Pcos diet book: how you can use the nutritional approach to deal with polycystic ovary syndrome.*

Harvard Health Publishing. (0AD). Foods that fight inflammation. Retrieved from https://www.health.harvard.edu/staying-healthy/foods-that-fight-inflammation

Hospital, B. and W. (2015, July 16). Understanding Polycystic Ovary Syndrome Video – Brigham and Women's Hospital. Retrieved from https://www.youtube.com/watch?v=Az9lWdqe-baU

How to Use Your BMR to Lose Weight. (9AD). Retrieved from https://www.livestrong.com/article/266994-how-to-lose-weight-with-bmr/

Karamali, m, Kashanian, m, Alaeinasab, s, & Asemi, z. (2018, August 31). The effect of dietary soy intake on weight loss, glycaemic control, lipid profiles and biomarkers of inflammation and oxidative stress in women with polycystic ovary syndrome: a randomised clinical trial. Retrieved September 3, 2019, from https://www.ncbi.nlm.nih.gov/pubmed/29468748.

Lagroue, C. (0AD). Can Diet and Exercise Actually Improve PCOS Symptoms? Retrieved from https://www.self.com/story/pcos-diet-exercise

McCulloch, F. (2016). *8 Steps to reverse your Pcos: a proven program to reset your hormones, repair your metabolism and restore your fertility.* Austin, TX: Greenleaf Book Group Press.

McMacken, M., & Shah, S. (2017, May). A plant-based diet for the prevention and treatment of type 2 diabetes. Retrieved September 3, 2019, from https://www.ncbi.nlm.nih.gov/pmc/articles/PMC5466941/.

Morris, A., & Rossiter, M. (2011). *Anti-inflammation diet for dummies.*

Orlov, A. (2017, October 3). How to Calculate Your BMR (And Why It Matters). Retrieved from https://dailyburn.com/life/health/how-to-calculate-bmr/

Prakash, S. (2018, December 1). PCOS: A lifestyle disorder. Retrieved from https://www.telegraphindia.com/health/pcos-a-lifestyle-disorder/cid/1677239

Rose, H. (2014). *Heather How to beat Pcos Naturally and Regain A healthy and fertile life now. A simple guide on Pcos DIet and EXercises to ConPCOS Permanently today.* Yap Kee Chong.

Stevens, P. (2016). *Pcos Diet Plan: The Ultimate Guide To Unlocking Polycystic Ovaries With Pcos Diet*

As A Pcos Treatment Approach That Correct Insulin Resistance Today.

Watson, K. (2018, April 6). 30 Natural Ways to Help Treat Polycystic Ovary Syndrome (PCOS). Retrieved from 30 Natural Ways to Help Treat Polycystic Ovary Syndrome (PCOS)

What Does Zinc Have to Do with PCOS? A Lot! (2019, February 5). Retrieved from https://www.pcosnutrition.com/zinc-for-pcos/

Made in the USA
Monee, IL
29 August 2023